ALLERGIES

Allergies

The Complete Guide to Diagnosis, Treatment, and Daily Management

Stuart H. Young, M.D.
Bruce S. Dobozin, M.D.
Margaret Miner
and the Editors of Consumer Reports Books

Consumer Reports Books
A Division of Consumers Union

Yonkers, New York

Copyright © 1991 by Stuart Young, Bruce Dobozin, and Margaret Miner
Published by Consumers Union of United States, Inc., Yonkers, New York
10703.

Library of Congress Cataloging-in-Publication Data
Allergies / Stuart Young . . . [et al.].
p. cm.
Includes index.
ISBN 0-89043-362-3
1. Allergy—Popular works.   I. Young, Stuart, 1938–
RC584.A344   1992
616.97—dc20   91-40481
                                                                CIP

Design by Susan Hood
Drawings by Mary E. Miner

First printing, February 1992
Manufactured in the United States of America

Allergies is a Consumer Reports Book published by Consumers Union, the nonprofit organization that publishes *Consumer Reports,* the monthly magazine of
test reports, product Ratings, and buying guidance. Established in 1936, Consumers Union is chartered under the Not-For-Profit Corporation Law of the
State of New York.

The purposes of Consumers Union, as stated in its charter, are to provide
consumers with information and counsel on consumer goods and services, to
give information on all matters relating to the expenditure of the family income,
and to initiate and to cooperate with individual and group efforts seeking to
create and maintain decent living standards.

Consumers Union derives its income solely from the sale of *Consumer Reports*
and other publications. In addition, expenses of occasional public service efforts
may be met, in part, by nonrestrictive, noncommercial contributions, grants,
and fees. Consumers Union accepts no advertising or product samples and is
not beholden in any way to any commercial interest. Its Ratings and reports
are solely for the use of the readers of its publications. Neither the Ratings nor
the reports nor any Consumers Union publications, including this book, may
be used in advertising or for any commercial purpose. Consumers Union will
take all steps open to it to prevent such uses of its materials, its name, or the
name of *Consumer Reports.*

Dedication

To my father, Julius, who passed away during the writing of this book. He taught me the principles by which I live. To my mother, Norma, and my sister, Diane Amar, who are guiding lights to me. Special thanks to Devorah Sperber for being here. —B.S.D.

To my wife, parents, and family, with love and gratitude.

—S.H.Y.

Contents

Contents

20 The Future 265

Introduction

Allergy medicine is one of the more personal branches of medicine, requiring good communication and understanding between physician and patient. A conscientious allergy specialist devotes substantial time to taking a patient's history and asking follow-up questions as tests and treatment are undertaken.

We allergists are among the few medical specialists who still occasionally visit a patient's home. The purpose, typically, is not to administer therapy but rather to search for some undetected allergen causing the patient to become sick. The culprit may be an antique chair stuffed with horsehair, a moldy closet, an obscure patch of ragweed, or any of a myriad of other possible causes that are all too easy to miss.

Allergists tend to have more than average empathy with their patients, because many of us who work in this field of medicine suffer from allergies and related disorders ourselves.

In my case, when I was about seven years old I developed terrible sinus headaches. They were painful enough to make me cry, and when they first occurred my parents were sure that I had a brain tumor. At that age, I didn't know a thing about brain tumors, but I was frightened anyway.

We were all relieved to find out that the headaches were actually caused by an allergic reaction to ragweed pollen. Like most children, I wasn't enthusiastic about the treatment—allergy shots—but I had to admit desensitizing me to the pollen helped a great deal. Summer and fall became far more enjoyable.

Dr. Bruce Dobozin, my colleague and the co-author of this book, was lucky enough to escape difficulties until he was in medical school, when he developed mild allergic asthma.

As anyone who has suffered from allergies knows, they are not among medicine's more glamorous disorders. The general public tends to dismiss allergy symptoms as minor annoyances. However, the patient may be seriously disabled. Asthma, particularly in children, can be devastating. A child who can't run without gasping or who can't breathe in a country meadow is missing out on life, and is often anxious and sad as well as sick. But today we can almost always get these youngsters back to normal health, even to athletic prowess.

In the past 20 years, we have learned a great deal about how allergies arise and we have developed more precise, effective diagnostic tests as well as better treatments. For example, we used to think that house dust, generically, caused allergy symptoms in some people. We know now that the culprit is actually a little creature called a dust mite. (The allergen is in the mite's feces.) Treatment with desensitizing serum is effective, as are measures to reduce the mite population in one's home environment.

In the treatment of asthma, the new steroid medications that can be inhaled work rapidly and well, while avoiding some of the undesirable side effects of oral steroids. Improved, non-soporific antihistamines now make it possible for some patients to get 24-hour relief from allergy symptoms, without worrying that drowsiness will make driving or other hazardous activities excessively dangerous.

As a means of communication with patients, most allergists hand out literature on the various types of allergies and their causes and treatment. Doctors also try to anticipate questions that patients may have. But allergies are more complex than most people realize; allergic reactions may be mild and intermittent, like occasional hay fever, or severe and even life-threatening, like an anaphylactic reaction to a bee sting, or a penicillin allergy, or a serious asthma attack triggered by an allergic condition.

For the person who wants a good general understanding of allergies and their treatment, something more than office literature is needed. To cover the relevant material requires not just a series of pamphlets, but a book.

We decided to write this book because of the lack of a comprehensive basic text for the general reader that we could recommend to patients who wanted more information. We particularly wanted to offer a text as free as possible of ideological bias. Perhaps because allergies are so complex and affect so many people—at least 50 million U.S. residents—they have been blamed for just about every imaginable disorder, from malaise and headaches to fatigue and hyperactivity. Responsible allergists in recent years have had to sort through a plethora of speculative theories and questionable treatments, some worthy of further research, others clearly fraudulent.

Our intention is to describe accepted scientific and medical practice and treatment, discuss those lines of speculation that may prove fruitful in the future, and warn against undertaking tests and treatments based on unproven or disproven claims.

In planning and writing the book, we aimed to provide information in as useful a form as possible. We do not expect readers to go through the text straight from beginning to end. Most people quite naturally tend to look up the symptoms or treatments with which they are most concerned. We have therefore tried to make each section as self-contained as possible and to refer readers to other relevant chapters as necessary.

The purpose of this book is to give you, the reader, information on what we know today about the causes and treatments of allergies, so that you do not suffer unnecessarily and, equally important, do not spend time and money on useless tests and treatments or on doctors who take advantage of your credulity. We hope you will benefit from the information in this book, written from our lifelong experience with allergies—from both sides of the doctor's desk.

—Stuart H. Young, M.D.

1

Allergy: What Is It?

Allergy afflicts millions of people worldwide, including about 50 million in the United States. If you sniffle in the summertime or sneeze when you clean house, you may be "allergic."

Many snifflers and sneezers go through life more or less contentedly without seeking a definitive diagnosis or medical treatment. Their symptoms just don't bother them much. But for many others, allergies seriously interfere with their ability to enjoy life and get their work done. These people usually want some kind of treatment, if only an over-the-counter remedy. For a few patients, allergy is a serious, even dangerous condition that requires expert medical attention and constant vigilance to prevent a life-threatening allergic reaction.

As common as allergies are, however, they are not always easy to diagnose. The first step is to find out whether your symptoms are caused by an allergy or some other problem, such as a chronic respiratory or intestinal infection.

Most patients visit an allergy doctor with one or more of the following kinds of complaints:

• Nasal and respiratory symptoms of the sort usually associated with a head cold or hay fever—that is, runny nose, sneezing, watery eyes, sinus headaches (pain in the forehead).
• Wheezing (especially on exhaling), shortness of breath, chest tightness, difficulty in exhaling completely. These are typical symptoms of asthma, but may be caused by other conditions as

well. Asthma is often but not always associated with allergy.
• Itchy hives or rashes, or other skin irritations. The patient
may suspect a food allergy or skin sensitivity to some chemical
substance, such as suntan lotion.
• Diarrhea or nausea. Food allergies are often suspected by the
patient.
• Headache, irritability, fatigue, malaise. The patient may feel
that a food or something in the air at home or in the office is
causing the problem.

It's ordinarily much easier to find the causes of the symptoms
at the top of the list than of those toward the end. In fact, until
recently, patients suffering from fatigue, headaches, or jumpiness probably would not have thought of coming to an allergist. In the past few years, however, there has been considerable
speculation that a wide range of ills may be caused by allergy or
allergylike sensitivities and intolerances.

Some physicians (identified as "clinical ecologists") diagnose
and treat an extraordinary number of so-called allergies. As a
consumer, you should be wary of any doctor who regularly de-
tects extremely unusual allergies, such as allergies to all synthetic
materials or to many different kinds of foods. Such a doctor
may be relying more on speculation than science. In particular,
watch out for so-called cytotoxic testing; it does not work. (See
chapter 19.)

Luckily, most allergy sufferers report symptoms and histories
that fit a common pattern, and a doctor who asks the right questions can quickly make a pretty shrewd guess as to the identity
of the guilty allergen or allergens. Normally, it does not take
long to confirm the diagnosis and begin treatment.

The chances that you are allergic to something are increased
if one or both of your parents are or were allergic. There are
certain physical signs that indicate allergy; for example, swollen,
darkened eyes (almost like black eyes) are likely to appear in
allergies affecting the respiratory tract. Also, many patients have
noticed a pattern to their symptoms that suggests an allergy is
at work. This is often the case when the symptoms are seasonal,
or are related to a particular locale, or are associated with eating
certain foods. By trial and error, a patient may have found that
antihistamines (which block allergic reactions) are helpful when

he or she feels sick. If antihistamines help, the ailment is probably caused by an allergy.

The Allergic Reaction

Allergic reactions are triggered by the immune system, the complex system that recognizes and combats outside substances or organisms that get into the body. An allergy is a mistake by the immune system. The system reacts vigorously, even violently, to some harmless substance.

For example, a family gets a cat, and everyone is fine except for one daughter, Alice, who after a few weeks or months begins to sneeze and wheeze anytime she is around the cat. Alice, it turns out, is sensitive to cat dander.

The dander from one cat is essentially harmless. Nevertheless, Alice gets sick because her body reacts to a few specks of dander as if this were an invasion of pneumonia bacteria or some other dangerous substance.

When pneumonia bacteria arrive in the nose or throat, a whole series of defensive reactions occurs. Antibodies, which are special proteins produced by the immune system, attach themselves to the outer surface of the bacteria. A war on several fronts ensues, with the antibodies attacking the bacteria directly and also attracting inflammatory cells (white blood cells) to catch, engulf, and destroy the bacteria.

In an allergy reaction a very similar battle occurs. But in allergy, the antibodies are assisted by mast cells and, to a lesser degree, by basophils. Mast cells are found in connective tissue throughout the body, especially near small blood vessels. Basophils, a type of white blood cell, are found in the blood; they also exit the small blood vessels and congregate where invading molecules are present.

Mast cells and basophils are defensive cells that resemble mobile grenades packed with histamine and related substances. When an antibody is attached both to an "enemy" molecule (allergen) and to a mast cell or basophil, this signals the cell to set off an explosion of histamine and other substances, which together are chemical mediators of the allergy reaction. These cause swelling, heat, and often itching.

Allergies

An immune system reaction of this sort is pretty hard on the person being protected. The patient coughs, sniffles, and feels miserable.

Of course, when it is pneumonia that the antibodies are fighting, the uncomfortable symptoms and the harm to the tissues are well worth it, since the result is the destruction of these menacing bacteria. But when a similar war is waged against cat dander, as happens in some allergic people, it serves no purpose and is potentially dangerous. In fact, the term *allergy* was invented in 1906 by two physicians, Clemens von Pirquet and Bela Schick, who were struggling to understand sudden, unexpected deaths among patients who had received immunization injections against diphtheria, a frequently fatal disease. *Allergy* means, roughly, "altered reaction," and the doctors coined the word to refer to unusual, occasionally fatal reactions to the shots.

IgE

Unbeknownst to the doctors, some of their patients were allergy-prone individuals in whom a particular kind of antibody was likely to cause serious problems. Chemically, all antibodies are categorized as immunoglobulins. One type of immunoglobulin, called immunoglobulin E (or IgE, for short), is capable of binding to a molecule of cat dander or pollen or the like and binding at the same time to a mast cell or basophil. In the case of the reactions to diphtheria shots, the IgE antibodies were binding to molecules in the horse serum used in the immunizations.

This IgE, racing off to war for no good reason, is the culprit in allergic reactions. It was detected only in the 1960s, but for several decades scientists had correctly assumed it was there, causing all kinds of trouble for allergic people.

Strictly speaking, an allergic reaction is one produced by IgE antibodies (or sometimes by another related type of immunoglobulin, IgG subclass 4). *Allergy medicine,* however, is often defined more widely to include all disorders of the immune system that involve a heightened sensitivity to substances. Nevertheless, the distinction between being allergic to something and simply having a poor tolerance to it can be extremely important.

You may be sensitive to or intolerant of some substances, and react badly to them, without being allergic. The distinction may be of no practical importance, since you must avoid the substance in any case, but sometimes the distinction makes an enormous difference. If you are intolerant of penicillin, for example, it may give you diarrhea. But if you are allergic to it, it may kill you. (See chapter 8.)

Allergens Get Around

An antigen is any foreign substance capable of causing an immune-system reaction that produces antibodies. An allergen is a special kind of antigen that causes an allergic reaction. Common allergens include animal dander, pollen, bee venom, mold spores, and various foods and drugs, such as peanuts and penicillin.

Allergens are invaders. To affect their victims, they must find a way into the body. It is not easy to enter through the skin (including the lining of the eyes—the conjunctiva), which offers pretty good protection. Molecules of an allergen—say, cat dander—in contact with the skin usually have a limited, local effect, if any. You may get a rash and feel itchy. Various chemicals, however, can penetrate the skin and travel through the body. For example, an antibiotic cream used topically may sensitize you, causing the production of allergy antibodies. If you later take the drug orally, you may experience an allergic reaction in the form of a rash or fever or other symptoms.

The respiratory and alimentary tracts are much better ports of entry for allergens. Substances breathed in or swallowed may affect the entire respiratory tract (from nose to lungs) or alimentary tract (from lips and mouth to intestines). Ragweed pollen, for example, breathed in through the nose of someone sensitive to it, causes hay fever or, if it reaches the lungs, may cause an asthma attack. Animal dander can also provoke asthma as well as hay fever–like complaints.

This is because allergen molecules can escape the systems by which they enter, traveling widely in the body via the bloodstream. Thus, an allergen in food may activate mast cells in the skin, causing hives or a rash. Moreover, the histamine and other chemicals produced in an allergic response can cause a general, widespread reaction.

Often people overlook this traveling habit of allergens and look for local causes of symptoms. For example, if a baby has a rash, the parents often guess that the baby is sensitive to soap

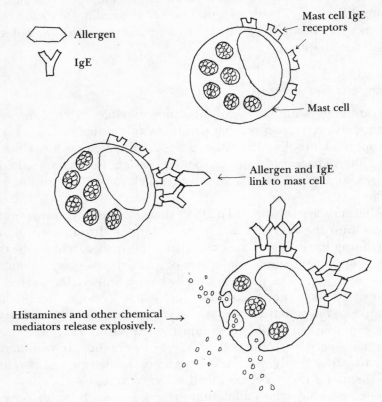

Mechanism of an Allergic Reaction

used in the wash. This may be true. But it is equally likely that the baby is allergic to milk. A baby with milk allergy will often also get diarrhea, a sign that the allergen is indeed in the alimentary tract.

In rare cases, an allergen can cause problems in remote organs, including the liver and kidneys. A patient at a large metropolitan hospital, who had been receiving penicillin for strep throat, developed fever, a rash, and blood in the urine. This kidney failure was evidently associated with an allergic sensitivity to penicillin. The penicillin was stopped, and prednisone (a steroid drug used to reduce swelling and suppress the reaction of the immune system in allergy reactions) was administered. The kidneys returned to normal function.

Treating Allergies

Supermarkets and drugstores carry dozens of medicines for treating allergies, including antihistamines and decongestants to be taken orally or as nasal sprays. With many allergies—particularly those that are seasonal or sporadic, and also mild—you can safely endure most of the more common symptoms or treat them with over-the-counter medications. However, it is also important to know when it may not be safe to use these over-the-counter drugs. For all but the mildest symptoms, we recommend that you consult a doctor before starting to medicate yourself for allergies, although that doctor need not be an allergist. A conscientious family physician may also be able to provide a more cost-effective and medically effective treatment than you can manage by buying over the counter. And a physician will be able to warn you if there is any reason why you should not take a particular drug. You may also want to know how to keep a mild allergy in check so that you avoid major flare-ups in the future.

Of course, you should not medicate yourself if you know or suspect that you have any important medical problem, such as heart disease, circulatory disease, kidney or liver disease, diabetes, or any serious chronic condition.

Finally, do not try to treat a child or a person over seventy years old with over-the-counter medicines except with careful medical monitoring. Both young and old often experience unusual reactions to drugs.

2

A Brief Overview of Allergic Diseases

Allergic diseases include those diseases caused directly by an allergy and those that result indirectly from allergy. For example, an ear infection may arise as a result of chronic hay fever, especially in children. (In youngsters, the immature Eustachian tube is more open, allowing material from the back of the nose and the throat to enter the ear.) Here is a list of the most common allergic diseases:

• Allergic rhinitis includes hay fever, mold and dust allergies, and other allergies affecting the respiratory tract. Sniffling, sneezing, and watery eyes are typical symptoms. At least 15 percent of the population of North America is affected with allergy of this type. (See chapter 10. Related problems in the sinuses, eyes, and ears are discussed in chapter 11.)

• Asthma, characterized by shortness of breath and wheezing, is a major health problem. Not all cases of asthma are caused by allergy, but many are or have an allergic component. (See chapter 9.)

• Food allergies range from acute, sometimes fatal, sensitivities to particular foods to mild reactions that are little more than a nuisance. (See chapter 7.)

• Drug allergies and intolerances affect some 10 percent of the population treated with drugs. (See chapter 8.)

• Urticaria, better known as hives, and angioedema, which is soft-tissue swelling, can be associated with a wide range of allergic conditions, including allergic shock (anaphylaxis). Hives are sometimes caused by food or drug allergies or sensitivity to bee stings. The so-called physical allergies, such as sensitivity to cold, can give rise to hives in the absence of an outside allergen. (See chapter 12.)

• Dermatitis, including eczema and other types of rash, often occurs as a result of allergies. (See chapter 12.)

• Anaphylaxis is an overwhelming, sometimes fatal allergic reaction. (See chapter 13.)

Hay Fever

The most common seasonal allergy is popularly called hay fever, although it is caused by a variety of pollens or mold spores that have nothing to do with hay. Typical symptoms are sneezing, sniffling, and burning eyes, occurring in the spring and summer.

Plants, trees, or grasses in the immediate vicinity of your home can be a major cause of hay-fever flare-ups, and it is a good idea to be familiar with what's growing near you. Some plants are far more likely than others to cause allergies. Your local hospital or doctor should be able to get you information on the most allergenic plants in your locality (see chapter 10). You can also follow the news on pollen counts through your local radio and television broadcasts.

Sniffles and Sneezes That Aren't Hay Fever

Respiratory symptoms that are not associated with the spring or summer seasons and that are worse indoors than outdoors are usually due to allergens around the house. The most common household allergens are animal dander, house dust (containing dust mites), mold spores, cockroaches, and feathers.

Technically, if these things make you sneeze or blow your nose, you suffer from allergic rhinitis, a term that also covers hay-fever symptoms.

Allergies

Sometimes a thorough bedroom cleaning or housecleaning is enough to cure allergic rhinitis (see chapter 4). But if the symptoms persist, or you find yourself frequently resorting to antihistamines or cold remedies to get some relief, then you should see an allergist.

Serious Respiratory and Ear-Nose-and-Throat Symptoms

Certain symptoms are suggestive of a problem serious enough that you should not rely on home treatment. See a doctor for diagnosis and specific treatment for any of the following:

• Wheezing, difficulty exhaling, shortness of breath, frequent coughing because of excess mucus, tightness or pain in the chest. One or more of these symptoms may indicate asthma, emphysema, a serious respiratory infection, or a heart disorder.
• Coughing up mucus that is discolored (gray, yellow, green, or brown, or even worse, bloody or blood-streaked). Such symptoms suggest an infection or lung disease.
• Coughing up mucus as small strings or plugs means that the mucus has been shaped by remaining too long in the airways. This may be a sign of asthma. (See chapter 9.)
• Persistent sinus pain, or chronic postnasal drip, or the production of discolored mucus when you blow your nose warrants a doctor's attention. The recommended treatment may be as simple as sniffing a solution of salt and water, but antibiotics may be needed. Sinus pain can occur in the forehead over the eyes or near the top of the nose and cheeks, under the eyes.
• Persistent headaches may indicate sinus disease or a number of other problems. Well-meaning friends may dismiss your headaches as "only" sinus headaches, as if they pose no risk to health. This is not so. Sinus headaches should be diagnosed by an expert. (See chapters 11 and 19.)
• Redness of the sclera (white) of the eyes without itching, or any kind of discharge from the eyes, may be a sign of an underlying disease of the eyes or of disease elsewhere, for example, of the joints or connective tissue.
• Persistent itching of the eyes, even if it seems just to be part of a hay-fever syndrome, should be checked with an eye doctor. A sensation that there is something in the eye, when accom-

panied by sensitivity to light, may be associated with an allergy but should be checked if at all bothersome to be sure it isn't something more serious, such as a scratched cornea.

• If you use contact lenses and have any of the above eye symptoms, you should tell your eye doctor. A variety of problems can arise from contact lenses, with a possibility of long-term damage to the eyes if they are allowed to go untreated.

• Ear pain or diminished hearing. See a doctor. Do not try to self-diagnose or self-treat.

• If you are a smoker of middle age or older, or if you have emphysema, diabetes, heart disease, kidney disease, or other chronic illness, do not try to diagnose or treat allergy symptoms by yourself, even those you may have had for many years. Your allergist and regular doctor should be in communication, in particular on the subject of effects of drugs you may be advised to take. Even if you do not have an allergist, it is important that you let your doctor know of any over-the-counter remedies you are considering taking for an allergy flare-up, even those you may have taken in the past with no problem.

Nonrespiratory Allergies
Rashes

Allergies can express themselves in a variety of itchy rashes, hives, and swelling. The cause can be allergens in the air, such as pollen; something eaten, such as watermelon or an antibiotic taken orally; or something in contact with the skin, such as nickel or cosmetics.

Atopic dermatitis (often called eczema) is an allergic rash that usually occurs without any allergen having been in contact with the skin at the location of the rash. It is typically associated with allergic rhinitis or asthma. Often there is a family history of other relatives with similar illnesses, and the patient with any of the three atopic diseases (allergic rhinitis, asthma, atopic dermatitis) tends to have at least one of the other two as well. For example, a patient with hay fever may also tend to develop atopic dermatitis; somebody with either hay fever or atopic dermatitis is much more likely to have asthma.

Atopic dermatitis is so troubling because the agent causing it may be difficult to identify. Furthermore, it itches, and repeated scratching can cause infections that over time badly traumatize the skin.

Contact dermatitis is a rash caused by contact with some allergen or irritant. The reaction may be relatively mild, as it usually is with jewelry containing nickel, or dramatic, as with poison ivy.

Avoidance is the key to relief of contact dermatitis. If the rash is relatively mild and you are pretty sure you know what caused it, treatment with antihistamine (orally) and/or an over-the-counter cortisone cream may be all that is needed.

The following kinds of rashes need medical attention:

• If the rash is eczema—that is, if it progresses to a thickening and scaling of the skin—consult an allergist or dermatologist.
• Any rash on an infant or toddler should be seen by a physician immediately. If that is difficult to arrange, at least call your pediatrician and describe the problem. Innumerable cases of so-called diaper rash have turned out to be eczema resulting from a milk allergy. (See chapter 12.)
• An itchy rash on the eyelids that does not respond to mild antihistamine treatment should get a definite diagnosis and specific treatment.
• A rash that follows treatment with penicillin, sulfa, or some other drug, or a rash that seems to be caused by eating certain foods, should be brought to a doctor's attention at once, even if the rash was mild and of short duration. Allergic sensitivity to drugs, food, or bee stings can progress rapidly to a dangerous stage, so that on your next exposure the reaction may be more violent. (See chapter 13.)

Hives and Swelling

Hives, or urticaria, are itchy swellings, something like mosquito bites, and always deserve attention, if not immediate medical treatment. Often people take them too casually. Hives need a professional diagnosis, even though in the end they sometimes must just be endured.

• If hives persist for more than a few days, if you feel sick when you have them, or if they are accompanied by swelling—for example, of the fingers or lips—see a doctor. Individual hives that last more than one day can indicate a circulatory disease (vasculitis). Normally each hive will disappear in six to ten hours.

• Hives may be the first sign of the deadly allergic reaction called anaphylaxis (see chapter 13). If they appear suddenly and are associated with rapid swelling of the throat, tongue, lips, or fingers and an all-over feeling of sickness, *you are in a medical emergency and must get help immediately.* An emergency shot of Adrenalin (epinephrine) may be needed within 15 or 20 minutes.

• Other kinds of swelling, whether or not the swelling seems to be associated with an allergy, should also be seen by a doctor. Swelling in the ankles and legs may be related to heart disease.

Nausea, Diarrhea, Aches, and Pains

There is a wide range of symptoms that are sometimes caused by allergies but more often have other causes. Stomach and intestinal ailments may be caused by allergies, particularly in infants, but more often they are not. The same may be said of headaches and fatigue. Arthritis is not caused by allergies, with the exception of certain drug allergies.

These symptoms are serious enough that you should see a doctor to determine the cause, although they are sometimes difficult to diagnose and treat. If you are being treated by an allergist or anyone else for the symptoms mentioned here and you are not getting better, consider getting another opinion, preferably from a physician with a different specialty.

3

A Visit to the Doctor: Examination and Tests

There are hard-sell allergists who claim to be able to cure everything from headache to pain in the toes, from stomachache to listlessness. They warn that you may have serious allergies without knowing about them, and suggest that a better life probably lies ahead after you have been thoroughly tested and even more thoroughly treated.

One allergist active in the Northeast mailed out a flier recently with a checklist of questions, including "Do you feel you are carrying too much weight although you don't eat too much?" For those who answer yes, and there are likely to be many who do, this physician offers a "metabolic allergy blood test" and a "personalized diet plan" that will take care of the problem.

If you feel that it is time for professional advice on symptoms that may be caused by allergy, we recommend a skeptical attitude toward dramatic promotional claims. You can ask your physician to recommend a board-certified allergist. The appendix lists organizations that provide information on allergists and allergy clinics.

You can also turn to people at your best local hospital or hospitals. A teaching hospital is often a most useful source, because doctors in a teaching hospital typically must keep up-to-date with the latest developments in the field of allergy medicine, a field in which new findings are occurring quite rapidly.

If you have a friend who's a well-informed hospital nurse, she or he may be able to suggest an effective, reliable specialist. Often a nurse will feel freer to comment frankly on a physician's work than another physician would.

A hospital's consulting specialist in allergy or the head of the department of allergy is likely to be competent. If not free to take on more patients themselves, physicians in such positions are able to make informed recommendations about other doctors.

Many people choose doctors on the advice of friends. It is certainly smart to talk to people who have been to the doctor you are considering seeing. But keep in mind that even a mediocre physician may have reasonably good results in most cases, so a favorable recommendation from a single patient may not mean much in terms of establishing medical competence. Nevertheless, in one area other patients may be a better source of accurate information than medical experts: how pleasant the physician is to work with. Allergy treatments often extend over months and even years—basically allergies are not cured, they are managed—so you want to like your doctor.

There are questions you should ask before committing yourself to long-term treatment with an allergist. Unfortunately, there is no one source for answers to all of these questions. Former patients may be able to answer some. Some are best asked of the doctor or the office staff. Some you will have to answer for yourself after meeting the doctor and the staff.

• Is the doctor a board-certified allergist? Depending on the severity of your symptoms, how long you have had them, and what success your family practitioner has had in treating them, you may be at the point where you want to be seen by a specialist. Your local medical society can confirm for you that a particular doctor who claims to specialize in treating allergies is in fact board certified.

• Does the doctor seem to be a good listener? Does he or she pay close attention to what patients report? It is nice to tell your friends that you are seeing the busiest allergist in the county, the one the local news reporters always interview when the pollen count skyrockets. But if the doctor hasn't the time for you, it's not likely that you're going to derive any benefit from being his or her patient.

• Does the doctor have someone to cover the practice if she or he is unavailable?

• Is the doctor responsive in an emergency? That means, for example, will the doctor work with the school nurse if a child has an allergy flare-up at school, or at least accept a call from the school nurse? Will the doctor arrange for an ambulance if a patient calls in with apparent symptoms of anaphylaxis?

• Is the doctor affiliated with a good hospital? If you are not familiar with the reputation of hospitals in your area, a good rule of thumb is to choose a teaching hospital, that is, a hospital affiliated with a university. A call to that hospital's physician-referral number will immediately confirm the doctor's affiliation.

• Are the doctor's office staff and telephone service pleasant to deal with? A good staff is essential to good medicine but especially to good allergy medicine, for here the doctor's assistants often do some of the procedures.

• Do the doctor's patients seem to function fairly well, despite allergies or asthma? The purpose of allergy treatments is to help people to function normally in the world. Some doctors are especially good at teaching patients to care for themselves; they encourage patients to live as fully as possible. All other things being equal, this is the kind of doctor you want.

• Are the fees in line with what other doctors charge? Though some top specialists do elevate their fees, medicine is one field in which it is not necessarily true that you get what you pay for. Sky-high rates do not necessarily mean you have found the most competent doctor.

Fee levels vary not only according to medical training, reputation, and years of experience but also according to geographical area, the personality of the doctor, the doctor's own financial needs, and so on. All in all, fees are not a particularly reliable indicator of quality one way or another.

If you do want to factor in cost when selecting a doctor, ask about charges at the outset of treatment. After all, many doctors ask their patients to demonstrate their ability to pay, and what is fair on one side of the equation is fair on the other.

Once the doctor has given you an estimate of what your treatment is likely to include and cost, you can then turn to your insurance company, which should be able to tell you not only which procedures are covered by your policy but also whether or not your physician's fees for those procedures are in the normal range.

• Finally, if punctuality is important to you, inquire about the average office waiting time. Many doctors overbook their calendars because otherwise they are left waiting by patients who show up late or not at all. So if your doctor does schedule appointments realistically, you should be particularly careful not to come late or miss appointments.

Service to Expect from Your Doctor

If you call your doctor with an urgent problem, you should be able to get an appointment promptly. If you are in the middle of an asthma attack, for example, you may be told to go to the nearest emergency room, preferably in a hospital with which the doctor is affiliated. The doctor should be able to meet you there or see you soon after the emergency treatment is rendered.

If the problem is not an acute emergency—say, you have experienced a gradual worsening of your asthma over the past week—a doctor ordinarily should be able to see you within a couple of days.

Similarly, if you have had an adverse reaction to a bee sting, a doctor should be willing to see you within several days to plan a diagnostic workup and treatment and to prescribe epinephrine (Adrenalin) for you to carry with you. After all, bees are more social than humans, and where there is one around there are usually many more in the neighborhood.

If you call in with a flare-up of hay fever or eczema, you may be asked to wait a week or so for an appointment.

Any possible allergy in an infant should be seen promptly by a pediatrician for diagnosis and treatment. The signs of allergy may include wheezing, persistent nasal obstruction, diarrhea, and rashes.

For a first appointment, especially a nonemergency, a conscientious doctor will usually allot at least an hour to get background information, do an examination, and conduct initial tests. The doctor may not be present the entire time, but between filling out forms and waiting for test results, the first evaluation might last as long as three or four hours. Use the time to evaluate the doctor and his staff, even as they are evaluating you and your condition.

Subsequent visits will usually be shorter—say, 15 to 30 minutes. If your treatment includes a series of desensitization shots, you may not see the doctor at all on these visits. But any time that you have questions, you should be able to reach your doctor in person or on the telephone to get answers.

A careful doctor should explain any test to be done and what to expect from medicines prescribed, including side effects. You should be encouraged to call if you experience certain specified side effects and to call about any side effects outside the range of what has been described to you.

Your doctor should have literature for you explaining how to avoid allergens that may be causing you a problem and how to medicate yourself effectively. For example, there are several wrong ways and one right way to use an inhaler.

A good doctor does everything possible to convey to the patient a sense of self-sufficiency. For youngsters with allergies or asthma, it is especially important that they not get the impression that they are invalids. The message they need is that they can lead normal lives. For example, a football coach who is willing to carry around inhalers for players with asthma, and who praises those players, goes a long way toward convincing youngsters that they can lead active lives.

Finally, the most important service you should expect from a doctor is that you get better as a result of treatment. This seems obvious, but it is sometimes overlooked. Whenever a course of treatment is recommended to you, ask when results should be expected. If you do not experience improvement on schedule, ask if it might be time for a new approach. If nothing the doctor tries seems to work, consider getting a second opinion from another doctor. Your first doctor may simply have missed something.

In one case, for instance, a woman living in New York had developed asthma. She was treated for a year without improvement and without getting a clear explanation of what had caused the asthma. At last, dissatisfied with this result, she decided to try another doctor. In taking her history, the new doctor noted that the woman's husband was a baker. Not only was he a baker, the bakery was below their apartment, and she often spent time there. Further questioning showed that when she was away from the bakery, she improved.

The woman suffered from "baker's asthma," a form of allergic asthma caused by a sensitivity to certain proteins in grains and flour. This had been missed by her first physician. Avoidance of the bakery took care of the problem. (See chapter 14.)

You should feel comfortable enough with any doctor to ask frankly whether he or she thinks you are seeking the impossible. But you should not be too easily talked out of your own convictions. There are, unfortunately, many examples of people wrongly dismissed by their physicians as misguided or hysterical, who have turned out to have genuine medical problems that required treatment.

To sum up, you are entitled to competent, courteous treatment and, in most cases, to treatment that works. If you are not satisfied with the results you are getting from your treatment, or if you simply do not like the doctor you are seeing, it might be time to consider changing to another.

Preparing for the First Visit

To make the most of your first visit to an allergist, ask how long the visit is likely to last. It can run two hours or more, so you may have to make arrangements to be free for that time. If you are restless because you have to get to work or back to a baby-sitter, you cannot get your money's worth out of this meeting.

If you are taking a young child, have someone with you who can help watch the child. Distractions are not helpful during an initial interview. Even if the child is the patient, it is advisable to have a baby-sitter on hand. You need to be able to concentrate on your conversation with the doctor.

Try to come to the first visit with as much information as possible concerning your medical history. There is a saying in medical school that 80 percent of the diagnosis comes from the history, the other 20 percent from the physical exam and laboratory testing.

You will be asked about major illnesses affecting close relatives, and of course you'll be asked whether anyone in your family has had allergies. It's surprising how often it is worthwhile to check with your relatives about this. Many times the questions jog long-forgotten memories. Among allergies, the atopic diseases—hay fever, asthma, and atopic dermatitis (eczema)—tend to be inherited and tend to occur together. So, if you have asthma, for example, and there is a question of whether the asthma is caused by allergy, it is helpful to know if other people in your family have had hay fever or eczema, even if you are sure nobody has ever had asthma.

If you are bringing a child for treatment, be sure that you know your spouse's family history as well as your own.

Be prepared to answer questions on your own medical history. People usually recall ailments that require attention every day, such as diabetes, but may forget to mention diseases that flare up only occasionally, such as ulcers or migraine headaches. You should have a complete list of any medicines you take regularly—over-the-counter medicines, even aspirin, as well as prescribed ones.

Try to recall in detail any previous treatment that you may have had for allergies. If tests, such as a pulmonary function test, were done, or X rays were taken, make an effort to get the results for your doctor. These records are yours by right.

If you have been treated for an allergy in the past, you will be asked how well you responded to the treatment.

Describing Your Symptoms

Think very carefully about your current symptoms. Arrange in your mind—or, better yet, write down on paper—the answers to the following questions:

• What is your chief complaint? Try to narrow the problem to the most troublesome feature—sinus pain, wheezing, runny nose, or whatever. The doctor will ask you about a whole range of symptoms, too, but it's helpful for the doctor to know right off what brought you to the doctor's office.

Be ready for detailed follow-up questions. If you have a cough, you will be asked whether you cough up mucus and, if so, what color it is. If you have ear pain, you will be asked whether you have run a fever in connection with it. If you complain of wheezing, you will be asked whether this happens more when you exercise or sleep.

• How often do you experience difficulty? Do the symptoms occur daily? Weekly? Seasonally?

• When did the symptom first appear? If possible give an exact date. At least try to give the time of year and how many months or years ago.

• Is the problem always of the same severity or are some episodes much worse than others? Do you tend to be worse off at certain times of the day or night? After exercise? After eating? Do you feel better on weekends or workdays? On vacation or at home?

• In what way does your illness interfere with your life? Does it affect your work? Your ability to exercise? Your ability to get along with people?

• What happened when the symptom first appeared? What were the circumstances? How sick were you? What other symptoms occurred?

• Do certain foods trigger your allergies? What kinds of food do you eat a lot of? Do your allergies get worse when you drink alcoholic beverages? (The answer to this question, by the way, is frequently yes.)

• You will be asked about your environment; whether you have pets and, if so, when they were acquired; whether you have down comforters and feather pillows in the bedroom; what you normally eat and whether certain foods seem to be associated with feeling ill; what soaps you use; what kind of heating system you have; whether your apartment or house is damp or if there is a damp basement (mold thrives in humidity); and so on.

Checklist for the First Visit

• Find out how long the visit will last.
• Collect medical records.
• Be prepared to answer questions about any family history of allergy.
• Prepare written or mental notes on your symptoms, especially when they first appeared and when they are most severe.
• If possible, arrange for child care if a child is coming on the visit.

Examination and Tests

A physical examination done by an allergist will be relatively complete, although it will focus on the head, ears, eyes, nose, throat, neck, lungs, heart, abdomen, and skin. It will ordinarily exclude gynecological or rectal examination.

In the physical, the doctor looks for characteristic signs of allergy as well as other possible causes of the patient's symptoms. For example, in the interior of the nose a pale gray-blue, boggy lining is characteristic of allergic rhinitis. However, a polyp or evidence of infection may point to a nonallergic cause of the trouble.

In one case, a little girl was brought in with a severe summer cold or possible allergy. The problem turned out to be caused by a piece of cotton that had lodged up her nose, causing infection.

X rays and Safety

X-ray procedures and some common tests ordered by allergists are described below. You should feel free to question recommendations for tests, on the basis of both cost and safety.

If you have had many X rays in your life and want to have as few as possible in the future, tell this to your doctor. Your doctor will probably not be surprised that you want to eliminate unnecessary X rays. If cost is a concern, ask what the price of the X rays or other tests will be and whether one or more of them might be safely skipped or postponed until the need for them has been fully confirmed. If you are generally healthy and the tests are not essential to the initial diagnosis, the doctor may agree that some can be deferred.

For patients with respiratory difficulties, chest X rays and/or sinus X rays are sometimes necessary. The X rays may be done in the office, or you may be asked to go to a hospital or laboratory to have them done.

If you have had X rays done recently, be sure to mention this, as they may still be useful. You have a right to copies of your X rays, although the office holding the X rays may charge a fee for copying them.

It is wise to keep a record of when and where X rays and other tests are done. The information can be useful later, sometimes years later. You can ask for copies of the X rays or test results, although it may be simpler just to record the findings, with the date of the tests and the name of the hospital or office where they were done.

Modern X-ray techniques, using a highly focused, low dosage of radiation, are much safer than the X-ray procedures of a generation ago. Exterior shielding still should be applied to protect areas not to be X-rayed. But actually, today, much of the unwanted exposure to radiation during X rays comes from internal scatter of the rays—that is, from X rays bouncing around among internal structures.

Everyone should have the abdomen shielded during the X-ray procedure, especially a chest X ray. Shielding is most important for children (male or female) and women of childbearing age. If a woman of childbearing age is being scheduled for an X ray, she should always tell her doctor if she is pregnant or if there is any chance that she is pregnant. If there is any possibility of pregnancy, nonemergency X rays should be postponed.

For sinus X rays, it is advisable to shield the neck to protect the thyroid gland. This is especially important for children.

A conscientious doctor will refer patients only to a radiology laboratory known to be safe and reliable. If for some reason your doctor does not recommend a specific laboratory (for example, if you are using an out-of-town specialist and you will be going back home for your X rays), ask your family physician for a reference. If you have no regular doctor, then use the X-ray facility in the best nearby hospital—again, preferably a teaching hospital.

It is difficult for a layperson to judge the quality of a radiology lab. Obvious clues such as holes in the wall, bumbling personnel, and X rays that need to be redone should alert you to the possibility of lax safety procedures. One might also be wary of a hospital or medical center near bankruptcy.

If you want to know more about the facility you are using, you can check the qualifications of the personnel. The physicians who read the X rays should be board-certified radiologists. Especially in radiology, which involves rapidly increasing risks if procedures are done improperly, the technologists must be properly trained, having passed a nationally administered examination and been licensed by the state. Proper positioning of patients for the X ray, for example, especially for sinus X rays, not only ensures clear pictures on the first try but also minimizes the hazard at each exposure.

A good X-ray facility will have a quality-control program that provides for regular checks of the equipment, although patients generally have no way of knowing if this sort of program is in place. Even doctors have no easy way of checking on a facility with which they are not familiar.

When are X rays needed? In general, whenever breathing is affected, it is important to have a baseline chest X ray (*baseline* means that the X ray will be used for the purpose of future comparison, as well as present diagnosis). People who smoke and are over 40 years of age should have a chest X ray every year or so. The chest X ray is called a cxr.

In allergy medicine, patients who have difficulty breathing typically are asthmatic. But it is important to do a cxr to be sure the diagnosis is correct. X-ray images help to distinguish between asthma and other possible causes of breathing problems, such as emphysema (in adults) or cystic fibrosis (in children). If the asthma reported is of recent origin or has suddenly become more severe, X-ray examination helps to rule out the remote possibility that the symptoms are related to cancer. In the rare cases when cancer is present, it is most likely to be in the form of bronchogenic carcinoma, but other benign or malignant types of tumor may affect the lungs. Hodgkin's disease or lymphoma (a tumor of the lymph glands) is also occasionally found.

Apart from the possibility of a tumor, allergists look for signs of pneumonia, chronic bronchitis, or a foreign body. In adults, especially smokers, we look for lung damage due to emphysema. In young children, we must consider the possibility of cystic fibrosis, which is characterized by excess production of mucus and collapse of air sacs in the lungs. Such a finding in a patient who comes in complaining of wheezing is extremely rare, affecting less than 1 percent of patients, and usually there are other symptoms that signal this trouble even before the X ray is taken. Nevertheless, it is important not to assume or rule out the diagnosis without viewing the lungs.

The cxr is also used to check for enlargement of the heart, although in cases where this is the cause of wheezing the doctor will usually have found other indications of cardiac involvement.

A cxr may also be recommended if a patient reports chronic hives and generalized itching. Patients with hives often find it strange that a doctor would ask for a cxr, but hives are occasionally associated with Hodgkin's disease, lymphoma, or other tumors (in descending order of frequency).

Allergists request sinus X rays when symptoms such as facial pain suggest sinus disease, or if there are nasal polyps. Sometimes in severe, unrelenting asthma, silent sinus disease is triggering the asthma.

Children under age ten who have sinus disease sometimes do not experience facial pain but instead develop a harsh, chronic cough. If no other cause for the cough can be found, a doctor will want to have a view of the sinuses. Very occasionally silent sinus disease can also cause hives. If a patient with hives of unknown cause also has some sign of sinus disease, then the doctor might ask for a sinus X ray to rule out sinus infection.

To avoid exposing patients to unnecessary risk, many allergists today ask for fewer and less frequent follow-up X rays than in the past. If the main symptoms are hives and itching, there is rarely any need for a follow-up X ray. For asthmatic patients, follow-up X rays can often be omitted unless the patients are on systemic steroids. In such cases, follow-up X rays should be done every couple of years or so. Of course, if the asthma takes a turn for the worse and doesn't respond to treatment, a cxr should be done to try to find the cause of the problem. Typically the doctor would be looking for some complication of asthma, such as pneumothorax (air in the pleural cavity—the space between the lungs and the chest wall, which normally contains no air and a minimal amount of fluid. This air prevents the lung from expanding). Mediastinal emphysema (air in the space between the lungs) has the same effect. The X ray also might show evidence of pneumonia.

Other Diagnostic Tests Your Doctor May Recommend

Sweat test for cystic fibrosis. To distinguish between asthma and cystic fibrosis, doctors will do a "sweat test" on children below age five who have asthma, on children below age ten who have severe asthma, and children age 15 or younger with nasal or sinus polyps or severe sinus disease.

The sweat test is painless, safe, and not expensive. It is based on the fact that with cystic fibrosis there is increased production of sodium and chloride by the sweat glands. In the test, the patient is given a drug (pilocarpine) to induce sweating, and then the sweat is tested for these salts. The test is far more reliable today than it was in the past, but for accurate results it remains important to use a good laboratory.

EKG. For most patients past 40 who come to an allergist with complaints about shortness of breath, the doctor may order an EKG (electrocardiogram; the "k" in the middle is a holdover from when the procedure was spelled the German way), especially if the patient has not had a recent EKG. The EKG checks heart function.

Pulmonary-function test. Most doctors who treat asthmatics or others with breathing difficulties have the apparatus to do pulmonary function tests right in the office. This test is done with any patient who reports a frequent cough or complains of problems with breathing.

Basically you are asked to breathe into a machine that can measure your lungs' ability to move air in and out. The measurements made are then compared to normal values for a person of your age, sex, and size.

One of the most important measures is FEVI (forced expiratory volume in one second), in other words, the amount of air you can blow out in one second. You should be able to blow out 80 percent of the exhalable air in your lungs in one second. This ability is reduced in severe asthma, although not necessarily in intermittent asthma.

The pulmonary-function test is often done before and then again after use of a bronchodilator (a drug that expands the bronchial air passages). A marked improvement as a result of taking the bronchodilator is one of the major diagnostic signs of asthma as opposed to, say, emphysema. Doctors also use pulmonary-function tests to assess how a patient is doing on a given medication.

It is very important to be aware that you may have bronchial obstruction without realizing it. To test for obstruction, doctors use a measure called PEFR (peak expiratory flow rate). For moderate to severe asthma, you can purchase a PEFR meter for use at home so that lack of air flow does not insidiously approach the danger point without your realizing it. The machine is essentially a tube with a rate-of-air-flow sensor. You blow into the tube, and the machine gives you a PEFR reading. (The machine is not expensive: it can be as cheap as $20.)

Urine test. Understandably, patients sometimes wonder why a urine test is relevant to allergies. Actually, hives are sometimes caused by a urinary-tract infection. Moreover, a urine test is an important indicator of basic health, helping the physician to rule out problems in kidney function, kidney infection, or in the urinary system generally that may be undermining the patient's health.

Blood Tests

Typically, any patient with allergies is asked to take a basic blood test (a CBC, or complete blood count), unless one has been done recently. This test, which is a count of red and white blood cells per cubic millimeter of blood, is a screen to check for anemia and other blood conditions and is a general index of health. It can also provide an allergist with a great deal of information that may bear on your allergies.

If you have symptoms of asthma, your doctor will check for an excess number of red blood cells (polycythemia). This excess indicates that the body is not getting enough oxygen from the lungs and is trying to compensate by producing more red blood cells to maximize oxygen distribution.

A differential white blood cell count, often done along with the CBC, gives the percentage of the various types of white blood cells that are present. In particular, if you are suffering from asthma or hives, your doctor will be interested in whether there is a high eosinophil count. Eosinophils protect the body from parasitic infections, and they modulate allergy reactions. Very high levels suggest an immune-system disease more serious than allergy; a parasitic infection; or exposure to a toxic drug or chemical, producing an allergylike reaction.

For example, a high eosinophil count is characteristic of the disease trichinosis (which comes from eating poorly cooked pork contaminated with *Trichinella* worms). Very recently extraordinarily high eosinophil counts were found in people who were taking dietary supplements of L-tryptophan and complaining of muscle pains and other symptoms.

ESR. The sed-rate test, or ESR (erythrocyte sedimentation rate), is a test for underlying inflammation. The principle is that inflammation changes the amount of proteins in the blood, causing the blood cells to clump together, thus forming a sediment faster than they normally do. If you have hives, a sed-rate test might be done to check for an underlying illness, such as Hodgkin's disease.

SMA-26. The SMA-26 (serum metabolic analysis) is a blood scan that measures a number of chemical substances related to healthy functioning of the kidneys, liver, and other organs. It also measures electrolytes (e.g., potassium) and blood sugar.

Complement. Patients with hives and angioedema (soft-tissue swelling) may show a deficiency in blood complement. (Complement consists of proteins that bind with antibodies; it is involved in many aspects of immune-system functioning.) Complement levels may also indicate whether the problem is hereditary or acquired angioedema—conditions that require entirely different management.

In very rare cases, syphilis is a cause of hives, but a blood test for syphilis would not routinely be done on an allergy patient.

If the problem is hives, itching, and/or swelling, a doctor is likely to run more tests if the patient is either over age 50 or under age five. Angioedema can be related to arthritic diseases in the young and old. Among older patients it may be related to cancer.

Alpha₁-antitrypsin. An important blood test for someone with severe asthma is an assessment of the level of alpha$_1$-antitrypsin in the blood. A deficiency in this protein is likely to cause early emphysema, which can masquerade as asthma. The deficiency may be inherited, so it is important to test for the protein, not only to treat the patient but also as an indicator of whether children or other relatives should be tested too.

The deficiency can be corrected by infusions of the alpha$_1$-antitrypsin protein. If this deficiency is found, it is vitally important not to smoke.

Cholesterol. For patients age 30 or older, it is a good idea to get a reading on blood cholesterol levels, even though these are not the immediate concern of an allergist.

Immunoglobulins, PRIST, and RAST

Immunoglobulin levels in the blood convey information on a patient's health with respect to allergies and immunity to infection. Immunoglobulins are proteins that function as antibodies, fighting infection and provoking allergic responses. They come in five classes identified by the letters G, A, M, D, and E, after the Greek letters gamma, alpha, mu, delta, and epsilon. IgE (immunoglobulin E) is the major antibody active in allergy. IgG, IgA, and IgM are more involved in fighting infection. There are also subclasses of IgG, the levels of which may be low in patients with asthma and other lung disease. The significance of this is not fully understood.

Two blood immunoglobulin tests that relate specifically to allergy are PRIST and RAST. Both are in vitro tests—that is, they are conducted with lab equipment rather than using the patient to test for allergic reactions.

The PRIST (paper radioimmunosorbent test) measures IgE in the blood. In this test, a paper disc is impregnated with antibody to IgE. The disc is first exposed to blood serum from the patient; then it is exposed to a control solution containing radioactive IgE (the radioactivity makes the IgE easy to measure). The more IgE in the patient's blood, the less radioactive IgE will be bound to the antibody in the paper. This is called a competitive test, because the IgE in both solutions is competing to bind with the antibody.

Elevated levels of IgE certainly suggest a possible allergic condition and warrant further investigation. But there may be other causes, such as intestinal parasites. Among severe asthmatics, a high level of IgE may suggest a serious disease, allergic bronchopulmonary aspergillosis.

One of the important advances in allergy medicine in the second half of this century was the development of the RAST (radioallergosorbent test) in the 1960s. RAST tests for allergy to a particular substance, while PRIST tests for the general tendency toward allergy.

Previously the only method we had for testing a person's sensitivity to a particular allergen was to "challenge" that sensitivity with skin testing using the allergen. This can be uncomfortable and, in some cases, dangerous.

RAST is done in vitro, exposing the blood taken from a patient, rather than the patient himself or herself, to a specific allergen and using radioactive markers to detect specific IgE antibodies to that allergen.

In theory, RAST is an easy way to find out if you are allergic to something: just give a blood sample for testing and wait for the answer. Unfortunately, the test, as is true of all allergy tests, is not entirely reliable, and the medical literature is not clear on which, if either, is more reliable, RAST or skin tests. A RAST produces few false positives but some false negatives. A positive RAST showing that you are, say, allergic to mold almost always means that you have that allergy. But RAST can miss some allergies and is slightly more expensive than skin testing.

For these reasons, many physicians do not use RAST unless there is some special reason to do so. (For example, the patient may have eczema, making skin testing difficult, or may be taking a long-lasting antihistamine, which will interfere with skin testing.) Others use RAST because of its simplicity, the reliability of a positive finding, and the convenience to the patient. They may follow up with skin tests if RAST tests are negative.

RAST when positive is definitive and when negative tends to narrow the field, sometimes making it possible to do fewer than ten skin tests, although up to 20 are needed in some cases.

But no single test invariably yields a reliable profile of a patient's allergies. Tests often must be backed up by other tests and considered in light of the patient's history and current symptoms.

FAST and MAST are variations of RAST testing using an enzyme, rather than radioactivity, as a marker.

Skin Tests

Skin tests are still extremely important in the diagnosis of allergies. In skin tests, suspected allergens, along with some of their near relatives, are applied to or injected into the skin. The allergist then waits 15 to 20 minutes to see if there is a reaction, called a wheal, which resembles a hive.

You must be sure not to use antihistamine prior to a skin test, or the result may be misleading. Some of the new antihistamines can stay in your system for up to a month, so be sure that your allergist knows exactly which medications you have been taking and when you last took any of them.

In skin testing, the allergen is applied to the surface of the skin (an epicutaneous test) or deeper into the skin (an intradermal test).

The surface challenge can be done either by scratching the skin and applying an extract of the allergen (a scratch test) or a drop of the allergen extract can be applied and a microscopic amount pricked into the skin. The latter (prick) test is preferable to a scratch test. With either test, a local reaction—a welt, or hive—may appear within 15 to 20 minutes. *But you must wait at least a half hour after the test in case the reaction is stronger than expected.* Most reactions just involve swelling and itching around the scratch or puncture. But sometimes the whole arm starts to swell, and Adrenalin is needed. An allergist will have Adrenalin and other drugs on hand to treat any dangerous reaction, should there be one.

The surface (epicutaneous) tests done by needle prick or puncture are very specific: if you get a reaction, you are almost certainly allergic to that substance, at least in the sense that you produce IgE antibodies to it. But this positive test result must be interpreted in the light of your entire history, especially when food allergies are being tested. Sometimes a positive result is valid, but not clinically significant; in other words, the allergen provokes a skin response but doesn't really make you sick.

Also, although specific, the surface prick or puncture tests are not as sensitive as we would like them to be. So it's possible for no reaction to occur as a result of the test, even though you may be allergic to the substance tested. For example, if you always develop hay fever in August and September, there is a good chance you are allergic to ragweed pollen, even if a surface skin test is negative. One way to check this further would be to use an intradermal test, which is far more sensitive.

The intradermal skin test, which involves injection of the allergen under the skin, has just the opposite qualities of the surface test. The intradermal test is very sensitive: if you are allergic to a substance, a reaction is much more likely to occur. But it is not very specific: you may not really be allergic to the particular allergen that provoked the reaction. In other words, the intradermal test gives more false positives.

Another type of skin test, the patch test, is done with patients who suffer from rashes diagnosed as contact dermatitis. The test is done by applying different chemicals to the skin under adhesive patches. The chemicals are often from a kit that contains the 20 most common causes of contact dermatitis. These are chemicals or materials found in jewelry, hair dyes, shampoos, medicinal creams, clothing, glues, cosmetics, and so on. The patches are left on for 48 hours. If you are allergic to what is under the patch, you will usually develop a telltale rash.

Challenge Testing

Challenge testing includes skin testing for common inhalant allergens such as pollen, but the term is more often reserved for tests for food or drug allergies. Essentially, this type of test in-

Allergies

volves exposing a person to a substance to determine if it will cause an allergic reaction.

Challenge testing may be called for in cases of a suspected allergy to penicillin or to a local anesthetic, when skin tests have been negative. With the patient closely monitored in the office or hospital, gradually increasing strengths and doses of the drug are injected or taken orally.

This procedure carries a relatively high risk of severe reaction, requiring immediate treatment. Food and drug allergies can be so violent that it is advisable to challenge such a response in the safest possible circumstances to find out for certain whether or not an allergy is present. (See chapters 7 and 8.)

Tests According to Symptoms

Exactly which tests an allergist is likely to request on the first or second visit will vary according to the symptoms you describe, your age, medical history, and other factors.

Unfortunately, there is no simple, inexpensive way to diagnose suspected allergies. Many tests are usually necessary, and even the tests do not always give the whole picture. Your own perceptions and your case history are also essential in determining if an allergy is present.

4

How to Avoid Allergens at Home

Once you have gone to the doctor and identified the allergen(s) causing you difficulty, the most basic treatment is avoidance. There is a great deal more you can do, of course, but you must avoid contact with the offending allergen or allergens, if at all possible and to the fullest extent possible, even when you are taking allergy shots or other treatment.

The majority of people with allergies need to reduce their exposure to one or more of the following common allergens: dust and dust mites; pollen from weeds, grasses, and trees; molds; animal dander and body fluids of animals (cat saliva is a particularly potent allergen for many people); and cockroaches.

In their offices, allergists usually keep literature for their patients on how to create an allergen-free environment. This material can be overwhelming if you imagine cleaning out the entire house all at once. Luckily, the job can be handled in stages, and often a few improvements in the home environment can bring significant relief from symptoms.

House Dust

Household dust is a ubiquitous indoor allergen (actually a combination of allergens) with an allergic potency that is much the same worldwide.

House dust is quite different from road dust, which is ordinarily merely an irritant, although at some times of the year mold spores and other allergens may get mixed in with normal road dust.

Good old household dust contains breakdown products of rugs and upholstery, such as down and various kinds of lint and debris, including kapok; cotton and sometimes cottonseed linters (short fibers that cling to the seeds); and animal (dog, cat, horse, cow, and pig) hair. Dust also contains tiny flakes of human skin, bits of plants, food remnants, animal dander, cockroach fragments, bacteria, and more.

Dust Mites

For many years, researchers were mystified as to why house dust appeared to cause similar problems worldwide. After all, cultures varied significantly in types of upholstery, foods, cleaning materials, pets, and so on that would leave traces in the dust.

The Europeans were way ahead of us in solving the puzzle, determining more than 50 years ago that dust mites were an important allergen. As early as 1920, W. Storm Van Leeuwen in Holland realized that mites in grain were very allergenic, and several years later H. Dekker in Germany discovered that the mites that live on human dander cause allergy. These findings, though, were ignored by English and American scientists until the 1960s and 1970s, when another Dutch scientist, R. Voorhorst, and a Japanese researcher, T. Miyamoto, established the dust mite's almost worldwide role in causing allergy. The tiny, barely visible dust mite is truly the global star of household dust.

There are over 50,000 species of mites, but the mites that most concern us here are *Dermatophagoides farinae* and *Dermatophagoides pteronyssimus*. (The term *Dermatophagoides* means "skin eaters," and these creatures thrive on their high-protein diet.) A third type of dust mite is *Euroglyphus maynei*.

The specific problem with mites is that, naturally enough, they produce feces, which at about 10 microns in diameter are exactly the right size to be breathed into the nose and other parts of the respiratory tract. (Ragweed pollen grains, at about 20 microns in diameter, are also in this size range. Breakdown products of these relatively large particles may be under five microns, and at that size they can enter deep into the lungs. A micron, by the way, is 1/1000 of a millimeter.)

Mites, having an appetite for protein, are more likely to be found in an environment relatively crowded with people and animals. (Recall that animal dander contains skin flakes.) They also prefer humid conditions (humidity of 50 percent and above). There are far fewer mites in high-altitude Denver, Colorado, where the humidity is low, than in sultry Miami, Florida.

Mites also like mattresses, rugs, upholstery, and natural materials of many kinds. They dislike plastic. Mites normally are not a problem in cribs, because of the plastic-covered mattresses.

The revival of interest in natural materials—down comforters, genuine Oriental rugs, English tweeds, and so on—has been a boon to mites. Many people, having invested in these popular products, find that they tend to cause allergy reactions, either directly (as in a sensitivity to feathers) or indirectly (as a haven for mites). Once mites have a foothold in your home, they are difficult to eradicate, producing a new generation every three weeks. (The females put out about 25 to 50 eggs at a time.)

Both mites and cockroaches can cause asthma, sometimes in a delayed but quite severe reaction.

Cockroaches

These clever but ugly bugs have been identified as important provokers of allergy reactions. Cockroach allergen is found in the body parts of cockroaches themselves, not in the feces, as is the case with mites.

More than 10 million Americans are estimated to be allergic to cockroaches, and about half of inner-city allergy patients react positively to skin tests for cockroach sensitivity. If these patients inhale cockroach allergen in a bronchial challenge test, they are likely to develop an asthmatic reaction. In homes, restaurants, and grocery stores that are infested with cockroaches, cockroach allergen is sometimes present in food.

Cockroaches like water, food leavings, brown paper and newspaper, glue, insulation—just about anything you can think of, they can eat or nest in.

Immunotherapy (allergy shots) using cockroach serum may prove to be helpful in reducing sensitivity to cockroaches. But the effectiveness of this method of treatment has not yet been fully evaluated.

Mold

Molds are primitive plants that lack chlorophyll and feed on other organic material, which they decompose in order to produce food for themselves. There are many thousands of varieties, and they are very adaptable, surviving both outdoors and indoors. It is the mold spores, which are tiny reproductive cells, that cause the difficulty to allergy sufferers. Among common molds are the black slime that appears in humid bathrooms, certain life-saving antibiotics, and numerous plant parasites.

People who get allergy reactions during humid or rainy weather (especially in summer—for example, when mowing the lawn), or when working in a damp basement at any time of year, are most likely sensitive to molds. The outdoor mold season is from spring to the first frost.

However, in temperate climates symptoms of mold-sensitive patients increase markedly after the first frost, because the frost kills all of the plants but spares the mold. As soon as there is a thaw, the mold will thrive on the dead foliage until the hard frost sets in. The indoor mold season may be perennial (year round), depending on conditions in the building.

How do molds get into our homes? The answer is blowing in the wind: millions of airborne spores settle on anything even slightly damp and organic. They grow on wood and fabric; they live in the refrigerator and under it, in the drip pan. They settle on house plants. They thrive in foam rubber. Molds enjoy humidity and are difficult to eradicate in a home unless the humidity is lowered. They can cause allergy, from rhinitis to severe asthma.

Pollen

Plant pollen is the notorious culprit in hay fever. Pollen granules can get into your home through open windows and on people's clothing. If you have been out on a windy day when pollen or mold spores are in the air, you may well transport the enemy in your own hair. A shower when the day's outdoor activities are over is often advisable. Otherwise, when you retreat to your clean, allergen-free bedroom you may carry a small cloud of allergens with you.

People who suffer from hay fever should pay attention to the prevailing winds and not settle down near an open window with the wind blowing in during hay-fever season. If you get rhinitis from pollen, molds, or both, be sure that your bed is not near a window on the windward side of your room.

Pollen counts are highest in the early morning. In pollen season, it is wise to leave the window closed and use an air conditioner from midnight to nine A.M.

Bouquets of flowers, unfortunately, tend to provoke symptoms in people who are allergic. A brightly colored flower is designed to attract bees and other insects to its rich package of sticky pollen. Putting your nose up to the petals and sniffing the delicious aroma can be like settling down for a picnic in a ragweed field. Flowers can be tolerated if you don't get too close.

As flowers begin to die, they get moldy, and mold is not something you want to introduce into your home.

Pets

Allergies to animals are common and very troublesome. Some people simply cannot give up their pets or their horseback riding or their farm stock—or their friends who have pets. And yet exposure to a dog or cat can cause a sensitive person quite a serious reaction. For such people, a combination of treatment and partial avoidance is the best treatment. In some cases, the allergy is just too strong, and the pet must be placed in a new home.

Allergies to cats can be particularly severe. There are people who cannot be in a house or apartment where a cat has lived in the past year without developing burning eyes, sneezing, and even labored breathing. Recent studies have shown that not only are cat hair and dander allergenic, but cat saliva contains a very potent allergen (and cats spend half their waking hours grooming themselves); the same allergen is found in the glands of the cat's skin, at the hair roots.

Almost all breeds of cat can cause a reaction in a cat-sensitive person. With dogs, however, sometimes one breed (not necessarily a long-haired breed) will bother a patient while another will not. Also, allergies to dogs occur less frequently. Dog allergen, incidentally, is in the dander, saliva, and urine.

The dander of cats and dogs can remain in a home, causing allergic symptoms long after the animal is gone, even years later. If you are taking allergy shots for sensitivity to an animal, do not stop the shots when you get rid of the animal. You will probably still need them for up to a year or more afterward.

Birds, Rodents, and Horses

Birds, and rodents such as hamsters and gerbils (yes, those cute little beasts are rodents), can cause as much trouble to a sensitive person as a cat or dog.

Pigeon and budgerigar (parakeet) fanciers run the risk of contracting pigeon breeder's disease, which causes shortness of breath, chills, and fever. These symptoms are dramatic enough that the person usually seeks medical help. But with one small parakeet, you may develop the same symptoms in a much milder, more bearable form. This is actually more dangerous, as you may ignore the discomfort and end up with a severely damaged lung.

Pigeon breeder's disease is a form of hypersensitivity pneumonitis, which is discussed in chapter 14.

Both birds and rodents are messy. Birds molt, preen themselves, and shake feather debris all over the place. Rodents kick up dust. Sometimes a young child in kindergarten or first grade may sneeze and sniffle if seated near a hamster's cage in the classroom. Before getting a bird or rodent as a pet for a child, try a few test visits of at least several hours at a time with the species of your choice. However, even if your child does not react, some children eventually become allergic to furry animals, and this could cause a problem in the future.

Horses are no longer part of most people's daily life as they were prior to the advent of motorcars. Also, horsehair is now used less often in furniture and mattresses. But people still ride or work with horses or use horse manure in gardens. And horses and horse products still cause allergies, which you should be aware of if you have contact with these animals.

Do We Have to Give Away Our Pet?

Every allergist is asked this question or one like it on a regular basis. Often the patient is near tears at the thought of losing the animal.

Some doctors feel strongly that a person who is allergic to an animal should find that creature a new home. This is certainly medically the best treatment. But getting rid of a cat or dog or horse, or even a bird or hamster, can be a draconian remedy when the pet is loved. And unfortunately, people (including children) who have not had much exposure to animals may not develop an allergic reaction for many months, sometimes up to two years. By this time, the pet may have become practically a member of the family.

If the prospect of life without your pet is too painful for you or for an allergic child, see an allergist about treatment and try to keep the animal clean and restrict its range.

You should not brush or wash a cat or dog yourself if you are allergic to it. Nevertheless, the animal should be kept well groomed, with a good wash or brushing once a week. The undercoat should be clipped or combed out regularly, especially in the spring.

If your local animal groomer is too expensive, the grooming is a good chore for a teenager or even a young child, whose rates should be more reasonable. The animal can be washed and dried in a bathroom and then the towels put in the laundry. Brushing and combing should be done outside the home. The brush and comb should be washed afterward.

An allergic person should not empty a cat-litter box or should wear a mask while doing so.

As for restricting a pet's range, the first step is to keep the animal out of the bedroom. Next, train it to stay away from your favorite chair or sofa. A cat or dog should have its own bed or one or two resting places of its own in the house. (With firm, consistent training—and strategically closed doors—this usually can be managed.)

If the pet has a particular chair or sofa it rests on, it may help to cover that piece of furniture with a sheet. Wash the sheet daily or at least very regularly.

Some animals do not mind being restricted to one or two rooms of an apartment or house for much of the day. If you live in the country, you may find that you can prepare quarters for the animal on a porch, in a basement, or in a garage or barn. But as a rule, an outdoor home for a pet is successful only if the animal has been conditioned to live outdoors from the beginning.

There is not much benefit to keeping a pet out of doors if you then weaken and let it in occasionally. Once the animal has spread dander inside the home, it may take many cleanings to get rid of the allergen.

Allergies

Check with a veterinarian or ASPCA representative or other expert on how to keep your pet safely (and hygienically) out of doors. People sometimes overestimate the hardiness of pets and lose them to freezing temperatures.

If you are at all sensitive to birds or to rodents, such as hamsters or gerbils, do not clean their cages.

After playing with a cat or dog or riding a horse, wash your hands or take a shower, and wash or clean your clothes before wearing them again.

Cleaning the House

Millions of people are mildly sensitive to house dust but do not need to take any special measures to guard against exposure. Others find that their reactions to dust are really troublesome, especially at times of year when they may already be bothered by pollen or mold.

How do you know if you are sensitive to house dust? An allergy may be indicated by a RAST blood test or a skin test. But simple observation may be test enough.

Do you sneeze and do your eyes itch when you are cleaning house or when you shake out a dusty blanket? Do you have trouble when the heat is turned on in winter? Dust that has settled in the system is blown through the air, and heat currents cause dust, dander, and mite particles to become airborne.

Do you have a severe sneezing attack when you change the bag in the vacuum cleaner?

Frankly, you do not need a medical degree to diagnose the ailment. The question is, what should you do about it? If your symptoms are mild or occasional, simply try to avoid exposing yourself to dust. Wear a mask or ask someone else in the family to help. But if you are affected more severely, and especially if you are asthmatic, you may need to take steps to reduce dust dramatically.

Dust Reduction

The first place that needs attention is the bedroom. People with allergies who can get a good six to eight hours' sleep in an allergen-free room often do quite well the rest of the time.

1. Change or alter bedding. The bed's mattress and box springs should be vacuumed and then encased in a zippered hypoallergenic plastic cover. To be extra safe, seal over the zipper with plastic tape. Mattresses not only attract dust mites, they often contain allergenic materials such as horsehair.

Companies that sell products for allergy patients offer a type of material that is plastic on one side and cloth on the other. This is much more comfortable on mattresses and pillows than all-plastic covers.

A person showing symptoms of allergy should not use feather pillows, a down cover, or wool blankets or mattress pads. When you change the bed, which you should do every week or ten days, vacuum the mattress pad or wash it, and wash the bedding regularly in water as hot or hotter than 140°F if possible. In addition, encase the pillows in hypoallergenic material or wash them with the bedding.

When you travel, take your hypoallergenic pillow with you.

2. Remove carpets and rugs. After obtaining hypoallergenic bedding, the next step is to remove any carpet or rugs in the bedroom. Carpeting typically is loaded with dust mites and is a major source for reinfesting the bedding.

If you want to try to keep a carpet or rug in the bedroom, it should be dry-cleaned or steam-cleaned every six months or so and then vacuumed every few days. Shaggy rugs are inevitably going to be very difficult to live with. A rug or carpet with a short pile or smooth weave may be tolerable, although vacuuming does not effectively remove dust-mite allergen from within the carpet, only from the surface.

Recently it was discovered that dust-mite allergen is broken down (denatured) by tannic acid, which is found in tea. A solution of 3 percent tannic acid (called Allergy Control Solution) is sold through antiallergy-supply sources for use primarily on carpets. Follow the directions carefully (including testing the carpet for colorfastness). A spraying should last two months.

An effective and safe acaricide (which kills mites in carpeting) has just been introduced into the United States. It contains benzyl benzoate, the active ingredient in the medication used to treat scabies, a skin disease caused by a related mite. Its trade name is Acarosan, and it comes as a moist powder. The powder should be brushed into the carpeting and left for about 12 hours, at which time a further brushing should be done to expose the powder to more mites. Several hours after the second brushing the carpet should be thoroughly vacuumed. This effectively kills mites and removes the mite allergen as well. Acarosan will soon be available as a foam as well as a powder. The treatment lasts approximately six months, depending on the original conditions. The foam can be used on furniture and bedding.

3. Clean the room. Now, give the room a good cleaning, and if you are allergic to dust, consider getting someone else to do the job. If that is not possible, use a damp or oily mop and damp or oily dust rags to keep the dust from flying up. Wear gloves and a surgical mask while dusting.

These steps are often adequate, but a very allergic person may need an even cleaner environment.

4. Clear out clutter. In the bedroom and throughout the house, reduce or clear out clutter—that is, dust catchers and debris such as pennants and wall hangings; collections of stuffed animals; neglected closets full of old clothes and dusty items on shelves; that ten-year supply of dust rags in the utility closet. Books should be in glass cases or should be dusted regularly. (Keeping books clean will lengthen their life, by the way.)

Suppose you have invested in Persian rugs or wall-to-wall carpeting for the living room. Luckily, it is not as important to get carpeting out of the living room as out of the bedroom. Try frequent cleaning, perhaps backed up with use of a mite-allergen-control fluid (tannic acid).

5. Change the furniture. The ideal furniture for an allergic person is Danish modern or something similar, that is, furniture made of sealed wood, plastic, and metal with a minimum of stuffing. Upholstered furniture with stuffing of animal hair, cottonseed, or kapok is likely to cause trouble. In humid conditions even foam-rubber stuffing tends to harbor dust mites.

The change in furniture may have to be gradual. But the allergic person should avoid musty sofas and chairs. Treat yourself to a modern recliner with a vinyl or leather cover.

6. Avoid heavy drapes and venetian blinds. Venetian blinds and lined silk floor-to-ceiling drapes grab onto dust. You are much better off with thin, washable synthetic drapes or curtains.

If you are not willing to discard heavy drapes or curtains, have them cleaned frequently. Venetian blinds can be vacuumed and also washed in the bathtub.

Drapes and blinds can be replaced by window shades (which are easier to clean). There are some rather elegant shades now on the market, including thermal shades.

7. Wash down the area. Wash down walls and shelves. Wash floors if possible.

Cleaning: Cure or Curse?

As you may have gathered by now, cleaning is sometimes unhealthy for the allergic person. Perhaps the only benefit of perennial (year-round) rhinitis is that you have a right to ask someone else to do much of your cleaning. Often it is best for the allergic person to be off the premises while the cleaning is done and for eight hours afterward.

The process of vacuuming fills the air with dust disturbed by the flow of the exhaust and by the movement of furniture. Also, fine particles of dust escape through the bag and the exhaust. The result is that, in the short run at least, you'll inhale more dust while vacuuming than if you just curled up in the uncleaned room with a good book. (Generally pollen and mite allergen settle out of the air in a few minutes. Mold spores and dander remain airborne much longer, but settle eventually.)

If the allergy-afflicted person is stuck with the job of housecleaning because there is no one else to do it, here are some protective measures worth trying:

• Filter paper is available to cover vacuum exhaust vents. If you are buying a new vacuum, you might consider a model that filters the exhaust. (There are also water vacuums that are supposed to be useful. But frankly, there is no evidence to prove that these machines really help.)
• A medical mask or dust mask can be worn while cleaning; the latter is available through dealers that specialize in allergy products or at a hardware store.
• Wear gloves to protect your hands while dusting or during spring cleaning. It is a good idea to cover up while cleaning, and wash your clothes afterward.
• To clean surfaces, use single-wipe dust rags. There are also mop covers that attract and hold dust. A damp mop is fine on most floors.
• To clean the oven, open all windows. In winter use a fan to

disperse fumes. If necessary, wear a vapor mask. These are sold by hardware stores for people who work with paints, wood strippers, and so on.

• You can reduce the frequency of oven cleaning by wiping up spills with a damp cloth while they are still hot. A self-cleaning oven gives off fewer fumes in the cleaning process than a chemical oven-cleaner does, but you still may need to ventilate the kitchen for an hour or more.

• To avoid rashes and other symptoms when doing washing chores, try a mild soap instead of detergent and oxidizing bleach (based on hydrogen peroxide) rather than chlorine bleach.

• Keep as few toxic cleaning products as possible in the home, and use them sparingly.

• One of the real hazards of housecleaning, whether or not you suffer from allergies, is the toxicity of many cleaning substances, such as furniture polishes, metal cleaners, moth balls, and pesticides for indoor plants and cockroaches.

Eliminating Mold

How do you know whether you are allergic to mold spores instead of or in addition to dust? You can be tested, but a few simple questions may indicate the probable answer:

• Do allergy symptoms flare up when you walk into a damp, musty house or basement, or a damp barn, garage, or church?

• Do you have problems when leaves fall, or when walking through leaves or raking them? Fallen leaves become moldy very quickly.

• Do you feel uncomfortable on hayrides? Allergy symptoms provoked by grass cutting or exposure to hay are often caused by mold, not pollen.

• Do you feel teary when you work in a greenhouse or sit among house plants? These often carry molds.

• Are your symptoms most severe on damp summer days? Very likely, you're allergic to mold.

Most molds in the home originate from outside sources but grow readily indoors in garbage bins, in food-storage areas, in wallpaper and upholstered furniture, and on bathroom walls, bathmats, and shower curtains.

Damp windowsills and bookcases are attractive to molds. One can find some truly spectacular growths in these environments.

To get rid of mold, you must eliminate dampness, clean up areas where mold is growing, and sometimes remove a favored mold habitat, such as a bathroom carpet.

• *Cut back shrubs.* If you have evergreens or other trees and shrubs growing close to the house, cut them back. Branches should not touch the house. There should be an 18-inch space between foliage and siding. (This will prevent the house from rotting, too.)

• *Check your house or apartment for leaks.* Put a sump pump in the basement if necessary. Look for leaks affecting closets and walls.

• *Remove old wallpaper.* Paint instead.

• *Check the bathroom for leaks.* In bathrooms, you may need to regrout or recaulk to be sure water isn't seeping under the tiles or tub. Be sure the bathroom is well ventilated.

• *Empty the drip pan under the refrigerator.* Clean out the refrigerator, too.

• *Dry damp floors.* Dampness in floors should always be attended to.

Mold can sometimes simply be wiped away, using chlorine bleach or another fungicide. Common fungicides include halogen products (such as Clorox), phenolated products (such as Lysol), and benzalkonium chloride (Zephiran Chloride).

Clean mold out of bathrooms or other humid areas in the home every two to four months, or more often if the mold visibly returns. But read very carefully the label on any products you use. Some fungicides are highly toxic. Windows should be wide open during cleaning. You should limit storage of these products, for seeping fumes do nothing to improve the air you breathe.

Crawl spaces and other inaccessible spots can be treated with crystals of paraformaldehyde for 24 hours. Close off the crawl way during the 24 hours that the crystals are evaporating. Then ventilate it well.

Paraformaldehyde will kill mold, but it is irritating and toxic, and the job should not be done by an asthmatic or other sensitive person.

A person who is allergic to mold should, if possible, hire

professional cleaners or exterminators to eliminate mold throughout the home. Make it clear that you cannot live with lingering fumes.

If you want to or must do the job yourself, one source of information is the U.S. Government Printing Office, Superintendent of Documents, Washington, DC 20402 for their free pamphlet "How to Prevent and Remove Mildew."

Technology to the Rescue

Humidity is essential to the survival of both mites and mold. Cockroaches do not like well-ventilated areas. Any significant air flow tends to make them move on. Therefore, dehumidification and ventilation automatically reduce home-based allergens.

Dehumidifiers

Dehumidification can be done with an air conditioner (an excellent solution, but only in hot weather) or with a dehumidifier machine. Correct venting and fans can also be helpful. For example, an exhaust fan is a useful tool against localized humidity in a bathroom or laundry room. A fan and vent in an attic or cathedral-ceilinged room can be used to get rid of heat and humidity from a fairly large area.

There is, however, a bit of science to getting the most from fans and vents, so you might want to consult a knowledgeable builder or architect. Libraries usually carry do-it-yourself books and periodicals that offer information on this subject.

The first step in undertaking dehumidification is to assess the extent of the problem. There are some obvious clues to high humidity, such as sweating windowpanes in winter or paint peeling off a house.

For a precise measure of home humidity, you can pick up a humidity gauge at almost any hardware store. A range of 40 percent to no higher than 50 percent is good. Humidity lower than 35 percent can make breathing uncomfortable for people with asthma and some other respiratory conditions, but generally low humidity is not the health hazard that high humidity is.

Do not overlook a check of humidity in out-of-the-way spots, such as a crawl way, attic, basement, or laundry room. Wrapping cold-water pipes with insulation will prevent them from sweating and decrease dampness in such closed-in areas. Storing firewood in the house increases humidity. Wood gives off a surprising amount of moisture as it dries out.

If you decide to buy a dehumidifier, use a reliable retailer who will take the time to help you determine what size machine (or machines) you need for your particular situation. From the physician's point of view, the most important thing about a dehumidifier is that it be kept clean (it should be cleaned daily); otherwise, mold will proliferate in the tank, causing more problems than the dehumidifier cures. One can actually smell mold flourishing in some dehumidifiers. Follow the cleaning directions very scrupulously. The machine should come with a solution that will prevent mold growth.

Humidifiers

In most parts of the country, through most of the year, humidifiers are not needed; levels seldom drop below 35 percent, and too much humidity promotes mite and mold growth throughout the house. However, depending on your area and your home heating system, a well-heated house can be very dry in the winter.

Some hot-air heating systems have a built-in humidifier, often little more than a container of water over which the forced air is passed before it circulates through the house. At times, separate humidifiers are used, especially in homes with antique furniture or valuable paintings to protect. Often humidifiers or vaporizers are helpful to asthmatics and others with breathing problems. Ironically, they also tend to distribute molds, bacteria, and pollutants that are likely to sicken the patient and everyone else in the place. If you have a humidifier attachment on your heater, or a separate humidifier, it is crucial to keep it clean.

For a number of years it's been known that standard humidifiers, requiring a reservoir of tepid or room-temperature water, foster bacteria and molds that are vaporized into the air you breathe. This can cause "humidifier fever," a flulike infection of the respiratory system.

Ultrasonic humidifiers were developed to overcome these drawbacks in the standard machines. The ultrasonic waves in the new machines kill off harmful microorganisms. Unfortunately, they also spew fragments of the dead microorganisms (often these fragments are allergens) into the air along with molecules of the minerals and gases in the water, including in some cases calcium, asbestos, lead, and aluminum.

If the humidifier is leaving a deposit of white dust on surfaces in the room where it is working, you probably have mineral-rich water. The white dust is made of tiny mineral particles.

There are a couple of different approaches to reducing the minerals and other particles spread around by the ultrasonic machines. One is to install a demineralization filter (filters should be available through the machine's manufacturer). The filters, however, vary in quality and effectiveness.

Another approach is to use distilled water, which has a lower mineral content, in the humidifier. But a study by the Environmental Protection Agency in the late 1980s indicated that humidifying machines filled with distilled water still produced about twice as many particles as would normally be found in the interior environment.

Thus, even with extra safety precautions, it's not clear that humidifiers are as safe as one would like. But if you are one of those people who cannot breathe comfortably in very dry air, then the trade-off is probably worth it.

There are also so-called warm-mist humidifiers, which do not distribute mineral dust, because as the water boils the minerals drop to the bottom of the tank. But these machines tend to promote mold growth as the vapor settles on surfaces.

Old-fashioned vaporizers, designed primarily to sit beside the bed of a sick person, are all right for occasional use (if cleaned after each use). But they cannot provide a general solution to low humidity in the home.

If there is a child in the home, or someone very elderly or ill, one must be vigilant to ensure that a steam vaporizer cannot be tipped over, causing a scalding injury.

By and large, it is best to use humidifiers of any sort sparingly. The health benefit is limited, except for infants with croup, who sometimes need a long visit in a steamy bathroom with a shower running. But in general, low humidity is not harmful to humans. After all, people with respiratory problems often move to the desert, where the air is very dry indeed. Your body has its own humidifying mechanism in its nostrils and airways. By the time air reaches your lungs, it is adequately humidified.

Cutting back on heat in winter ordinarily results in moister air. A pan of water on the radiator will increase humidity, but the pan must be cleaned every day.

Climate Control: Air Conditioners and Central Heating Systems

An air conditioner is almost essential to filter summertime air for those sensitive to pollen and other seasonal airborne allergens. It is also an excellent dehumidifier and thus limits the proliferation of dust mites and mold. The air flow discourages cockroaches.

Whether the air-conditioning is a central unit or a window box, the filters must be cleaned frequently, both for maximum efficiency and to prevent mold growth.

Central-system air-conditioning and heating can be equipped with electrostatic filters that catch smaller particles, such as dander, which may get through an ordinary filter. Electronic filters work by imparting a charge to particles in the air as they pass through the filter and then trapping the particles with an oppositely charged plate in the unit. These devices, too, must be cleaned often.

Electrostatic filters have one drawback: they may produce ozone, which makes asthma worse. This hazard can be greatly reduced by the installation of a charcoal filter in conjunction with the electrostatic filter. This has been standard practice by manufacturers in the United States for some ten years now.

There are filters that can be placed over individual outlet ducts of central heating and cooling systems. If you cannot find filters specifically designed for this use, substitute air-conditioner filters. Clean the filters once a week and replace as necessary.

Unfortunately, it is not clear that the filters available for home heating systems are fully effective. Ask for guaranteed specifications on the size of the particle that the filter will trap. Five microns or less is good.

Any air flow tends to disturb dust. If you have an air conditioner or hot-air heating outlet in the bedroom, try to get the room fairly dust-free before turning on the air conditioner or furnace.

Some forced-air heating systems come with a humidifying element to counteract dryness. This is double trouble: dust is kicked up by the hot air, and mold may emerge from the humidifying element. The systems should come with instructions for cleaning, and the cleaning must be done on schedule. Some people have the humidifying feature removed.

Allergy sufferers find radiant-heat systems, such as electric heating and hot-water heating, preferable to forced-air systems, which blow allergens and irritants all over the place.

Room air-filtration devices. Room air-filtration devices are sometimes recommended for people with allergies or asthma. A 1988 report by the American Academy of Allergy and Immunology suggested that such devices might be of some help in reducing asthma attacks, but the studies' results did not reach the level of statistical significance.

Various brands of air-filtration machines using HEPA and other filters are commercially available. HEPA stands for high-efficiency particulate arresting; these filters were developed during World War II by the Atomic Energy Commission to remove radioactive dust from the air being vented from nuclear plants. The filters are pleated to greatly increase the surface area, so they can eliminate very small particles.

Other types of air-filtration devices use electrostatic precipitators and ionizers to control dust.

Electrostatic precipitators have been accused of producing ozone, but tests of the newer filtration machines, with charcoal prefilters, show no apparent ozone problem. Unfortunately, the tests did not demonstrate much health benefit either.

A room air-filtration machine is one of the modern world's little luxuries. If you can afford it, it may be worth trying. But there is no hard evidence that such a device will really reduce allergens in the air. Some do a good job of reducing odors.

All in all, a professional housecleaning and the use of well-maintained air conditioners and dehumidifiers are the best proven allergen reducers.

Indoor Pollution

In a witty puppet show running in New York City in 1989, puppeteer Paul Zaloom imagined a house constructed of "4,000 man-made petrochemical substances." The puppet family that moves into "The House of Horror" does not survive the trial live-in period. Beset by chemicals in the rugs, furniture, and air purifiers, they develop symptoms ranging from rashes to psychosis.

The plot was drawn directly from medical headlines. Indoor pollution is a serious health problem. Moreover, the tighter we seal buildings to retain heat and save energy, the more acute pollution becomes.

People with allergies are often affected by small amounts of pollutants that others notice only in high doses. To give an example, some people are sensitive to tobacco smoke. A very little in the air makes them quite ill, giving them headaches and making it difficult to breathe. *No one should smoke, but especially not around a person who has allergies or asthma.*

Other fairly common causes of exacerbation of allergy symptoms at home are heating or cooking gas (natural or propane) and perfumed items, such as scented candles, air fresheners, and incense.

If you are sensitive to natural gas or propane, be sure that there are no leaks in your lines. For the lines that you can reach (those inside the stove and between the stove and the wall or floor), one test is to shake up detergent with a little water, wipe it on the lines, and look for small bubbles forming. The bubbles indicate leaks. But the best thing to do if you smell gas, even fleetingly, is call the gas company.

Some people are bothered by the small amount of gas that comes from a pilot light. You can put an exhaust hood over the stove. You can turn off the pilot light and convert to an electric ignition system. But you may eventually find that you are most comfortable with an electric stove.

Space heaters that burn natural gas, kerosene, or bottled gas should be vented to the outside. These heaters produce nitrogen dioxide and carbon monoxide, neither of which is good for your breathing or general health.

Some people do not feel well in a house or apartment building that is heated with oil or gas. Smoke from wood stoves and fireplaces can be troublesome, especially to asthmatics.

To reduce pollution from heating-oil fumes, vent the fumes from the basement by opening a window or a basement door to the outside (if there is one) every couple of days. Also, exhaust fans in the uptake lines will draw fumes into the chimney more efficiently. You can try air filters in the duct work. Have your chimneys cleaned regularly (a safety measure in any case). Lower the thermostat setting.

If none of these measures are satisfactory, you may do better with an electric heating system.

Painting and floor waxing can cause flare-ups of allergy and asthma symptoms. If this is true for you, have the job done by others at a time when you can be out of the house for several days. Working with water-based paint has less effect on asthmatics than working with oil-based paint.

Structural Pollutants

Some materials and chemicals built into home or office construction can cause allergylike reactions.

Carpet. One recently suspect item used in both homes and offices is wall-to-wall carpet. No one knows at this point whether the reported illnesses associated with certain newly installed carpets are caused by the glue, the latex backings, or the carpets themselves, but the symptoms include burning eyes, nasal irritation, and breathing problems.

The U.S. Consumer Product Safety Commission is currently studying adverse effects associated with new carpet, so if you have a complaint, call 1-800-638-2772 or write: Carpet Complaints, Room 529, U.S. Consumer Product Safety Commission, Washington, DC 20207.

Insulation. If you are buying insulation, you should check the product with a reliable evaluation service and with an informed allergist. If you are buying a home, have an engineer identify the type of insulation for you and evaluate it as you would a new product.

One of the substances formerly used in insulation and still used in other structural materials, such as some plywood and wallboard, is formaldehyde. (Also, from time to time there are reports of a flawed structural product from which formaldehyde escapes in excess amounts.) The effects of formaldehyde in relation to health and allergy are the subject of considerable controversy. At high concentrations, formaldehyde is very toxic, producing severe skin irritations and burning of the nasal mucosa (mucous membranes of the nose) and of the lungs. Formaldehyde is also carcinogenic.

The question is whether small amounts of formaldehyde escaping into the air in small amounts in the home or workplace are a health hazard. The answer is still not clear.

Formaldehyde, incidentally, has a fairly distinct odor. Your nose is not a bad formaldehyde detector.

Pesticides and Repellents

In recent years, the public has become much more aware of the dangers of filling homes with pesticides. More and more people, for example, are trying to control cockroaches by nontoxic means rather than with monthly visits from the exterminator.

Avoid treating house plants with pesticides and fungicides, especially during cold weather, when windows are kept closed. Try nontoxic remedies, such as washing the plants with detergent or alcohol. Throw out infested plants quickly so that they do not affect others.

Pyrethrum, a natural pesticide made from the flowers of a chrysanthemum, is related to ragweed. Pyrethrum is actually a safe, good pesticide—for everyone but certain allergy sufferers. To them it is a menace.

There have been reports of allergic and toxic reactions to heavy use of topical insect repellents containing 2,3,4,5 bis (which has been eliminated from many products now) and even the basic DEET (N, N-diethyl-m-toluamide). Be cautious in using these repellents. Do not spray them all over the head and body, and especially not all over a child. Use a nonspray liquid and follow the directions on the label. *Do not use products containing 2,3,4,5 bis at all.*

With respect to insect repellents, cleaning substances, and similar commonly used products, use your eyes and ears to follow health news. Always read the labels before buying a product for your home, and follow the instructions for use and disposal.

5

Allergy Medicines

Taking the commonsense approach of avoiding troublesome allergens is, as we have said, the first and most important step in allergy treatment. Unfortunately, it is not always enough. Sometimes avoidance is impossible: children with hay fever, for example, who want to play baseball and softball aren't going to find many pollen-free ballfields. If your fiancée owns a cat and you don't feel quite secure with the ultimatum "Kitty or me!" you may need medication to treat or prevent the symptoms you experience in the company of the cat.

People with severe or chronic allergies may need immunotherapy, or desensitization (allergy shots), to tone down their sensitivity to certain allergens. But symptoms that are mild or arise only occasionally can be alleviated with drugs, such as antihistamines and decongestants. Such medicines are sometimes needed even after desensitization.

Self-medication with over-the-counter drugs is often the first treatment an allergy sufferer tries. This approach frequently is effective and usually less expensive than consulting an allergist. But self-medication may prove unsatisfactory, and can be quite expensive as well, so it is best undertaken with a good understanding of the range of medicines available for allergy treatment.

Traditional Medicines

Certain drugs that relieve allergy and asthma symptoms have been known for centuries. The ancient Chinese used ephedrine, a stimulant that opens the airways, which is derived from a desert herb of the genus *Ephedra.*

Stramonium (jimsonweed) leaves when smoked may provide some relief from asthma. Atropine, which is found in these leaves, is the basis of the bronchodilator drug Atrovent. Unfortunately, jimsonweed can be quite toxic; when taken in large doses it may induce unpleasant symptoms, including hallucinations.

The key breakthrough in the pharmacology of allergy treatment did not emerge from ancient remedies, however, but from modern medical research. It was the discovery of antihistamines in 1942.

Antihistamines

Antihistamines available today provide relief from a wide range of allergic diseases, from hay fever to hives. The majority are not much help in treating asthma, but some of the very newest, including some still being tested, show promise here too.

Since the synthesis of the first antihistamine, diphenhydramine hydrochloride (Benadryl), numerous varieties of antihistamines have been created. Unfortunately, like Benadryl, many of these had unwanted side effects, especially sleepiness. This was a significant drawback to use of this type of medication.

Recently, however, terfenadine (Seldane) was formulated. It is a nonsoporific antihistamine; it won't make you sleepy. This is also true of a second new antihistamine, astemizole (Hismanal). These drugs make antihistamine therapy much safer and more practical than in the past. They are expensive, but the price will come down in time. As well, other nonsoporific antihistamines are still in the testing stage. So antihistamine therapy is a field in which both doctors and patients have to stay alert to new possibilities.

How Antihistamines Work

Antihistamines prevent histamine from acting on the cells of the capillaries (tiny blood vessels), nerve endings, and other cells that have histamine receptors. This action of histamine, working in concert with other chemicals produced by the body in response to invading allergens, causes allergy symptoms.

Recall that a double connection is needed to release histamine. The allergen molecule locks into a molecule of IgE antibody; the IgE is attached to one of the mast cells in the tissues lining the nose, lungs, or gastrointestinal tract. When the connections are made, the mast cell suddenly releases a large amount of histamine, along with other chemical substances, producing allergic symptoms. Histamine release also occurs when similar connections are made with allergen-IgE and a basophil, which is a type of white blood cell. (See fig. 1.1, p. 6.)

Histamine makes the capillaries widen and release fluid. This may result in swelling, such as hives. In severe reactions, a significant drop in blood pressure may occur. The histamine can irritate nerve endings, causing itching. In the gastrointestinal tract, it may cause increased secretion of fluids and cramps. And it may provoke tightening of the smooth muscles in the bronchial airways.

The histamine acts upon receptors on the surface of the cells that it affects. Antihistamines have a molecular structure similar to histamine and therefore can block the histamine from reaching its normal receptors. The antihistamine connects with the cell receptors, leaving the histamine molecules with no place to latch onto, like molecular losers in a game of micro–musical chairs. When the histamine can't get to the cell receptors, the chain of occurrences that makes up the allergic reaction is interrupted.

From this, you can see why doctors and pharmacists recommend taking antihistamines before your symptoms have appeared. You want to have the antihistamine latched onto the histamine receptors before the histamine released by mast cells can get there.

Try to anticipate the need for antihistamines. For example, if you are allergic to ragweed and you hear on the morning news that ragweed counts are expected to reach a century-high record, take your antihistamine. Don't wait until you're a weeping, sneezing wreck.

New antihistamines, being tested for use in controlling asthma, chemically stabilize the mast cells, inhibiting their release of histamine; and some new antihistamines cause bronchodilation (opening the airways).

Antihistamines are categorized according to the two different kinds of receptors that they act upon. There are H1 (histamine 1) receptors and H2 receptors. Therefore, among antihistamines there are H1 blockers and H2 blockers.

The H1 and H2 receptors are present on many human-tissue sites, including the very important capillaries (where H1 receptors predominate) and the lining of the stomach (where H2 receptors are particularly important).

There are many more H1 than H2 antihistamines—seven classes of them, in fact. The H1 antihistamines are particularly helpful in treating allergic rhinitis, or hay fever. But medical researchers are still studying the best way to use antihistamines in treatment. One fairly new approach is to combine H1 and H2 antihistamines to treat hives. In the past, only an H1 antihistamine was used.

Antihistamine side effects. The most notorious side effect of H1 antihistamines is sleepiness. This is not always an undesirable effect. If you are suffering from severe hay fever, a soporific antihistamine may help you to get a good night's sleep, but for daytime use the soporific effect can be a real problem.

Always check the label of an over-the-counter antihistamine or the warnings that come with a prescription antihistamine. As a general rule, be cautious about driving a car, operating dangerous machinery, or working in high places after taking such medication. It has now been shown that the nonsoporific antihistamines do not interfere with cognitive function in any way, whereas the other antihistamines always do, *even if they do not make you sleepy!* Your doctor can explain the circumstances under which it is safe to use any antiallergy medicine prescribed for you. Your pharmacist is another source of information, not only on prescription medicines but on those sold over the counter as well.

A special note of caution for those who drink or take tranquilizers: many antihistamines interact with alcohol and tranquilizers to depress the central nervous system, leaving the patient really groggy.

One of the advantages of Seldane and Hismanal, which are nonsedating, is that they do not usually interact with alcohol and tranquilizers. Although there are some indications that Hismanal is very occasionally associated with minor weight gain, the mechanism is unclear.

In general, most physicians today recommend extreme caution in taking any drugs during pregnancy. It is best to be stoic about allergy symptoms, other than asthma, until after the baby is born. The antihistamine PBZ (tripelennamine hydrochloride) is considered safest for pregnant women.

Antihistamines tend to produce tolerance. This means that a drug that at first makes you sleepy may later not do so. This can be a plus, but another effect of this tolerance is that the drug may not work as well to relieve your symptoms. At that point, your doctor might recommend trying another class of antihistamines to see if they are more effective. If you are self-medicating and develop a tolerance, try a brand made with a different class of antihistamine.

Certain antihistamines may produce what are technically called anticholinergic effects, such as heart palpitations, retention of urine, constipation, dry mouth, and nervousness. Therefore, one should be careful about using an antihistamine described as possibly producing such effects while taking any other anticholinergic drugs—for example, Bentyl, Levsin, and Donnatal, among others.

Consult with a doctor before taking an antihistamine if you are taking any anticholinergic medicine, antidepressants of the MAO-inhibitor type, or if you have thyroid disease, heart disease, or high blood pressure.

For seasonal hay fever, antihistamines work reasonably well. They are often used in conjunction with a decongestant, and many over-the-counter preparations combine the two, sometimes along with aspirin and caffeine.

Here follows a table on the antihistamines. Most of the over-the-counter, brand-name antihistamines are sold in combination with a decongestant. One asterisk (*) indicates that the medicine is available only with a prescription; two asterisks (**) indicate that it is available in both prescription and over-the-counter forms.

TABLE 5.1   ANTIHISTAMINES

Class/Type	Generic Name:	Available in:
CLASS ONE		
Ethylenediamines	Pyrilamine maleate	*Codimal DH; Codimal DM; 4-Way Fast Acting Nasal Spray; *Poly-Histine products; Primatene Tablets—M; Robitussin Night Relief; **Ru-Tuss with Hydrocodone; **Triaminic products
	Pyrilamine tannate	*Rynatan products; *R-Tannate products
	Tripelennamine hydrochloride	*PBZ products
CLASS TWO		
Ethanolamines (This class of antihistamines tends to have a more marked soporific effect.)	Bromodiphen-hydramine hydrochloride	*Ambenyl Cough Syrup
	Carbinoxamine maleate	*Rondec products; *Tussafed Drops and Syrup
	Clemastine fumarate	*Tavist products
	Diphenhydramine hydrochloride	**Benadryl products; Benylin; *Dytuss; also available in numerous sleep medications
	Doxylamine succinate	Contac Nighttime Cold Medicine; Vicks Nyquil Nighttime Cold Medicine

Allergies

Class/Type	Generic Name:	Available in:
CLASS TWO		
	Phenyltoloxamine citrate	*Atrohist; *Comhist LA Capsules; *Magsal; *Naldecon; Par-Decon; *Poly-Histine products
CLASS THREE		
Alkylamines (This class of antihistamines tends to be less soporific than the above.)	Brompheniramine maleate	*Allent; *Atrohist; *Bromarest; *Bromfed; Dallergy-JR; **Dimetane products; Dimetapp products; Drixoral Syrup; Poly-Histine products
	Chlorpheniramine maleate	Alka-Seltzer Plus Cold Medicine; Allerest; A.R.M.; *Brexin; *Cerose-DM; *Chlorafed products; Chlor-Trimeton products; *Codimal; *Comhist; *Comtrex; Contac Allergy Timed-Release; Coricidin; Dallergy products; *Deconamine products; Demazin; Dorcol; **Dristan products; *Drize; *Dura-Vent; *Endal-HD; *Extendryl products; 4-Way Cold Tablets; *Fedahist products; *Gelpirin; *Histafed; *Histor-D; *Histussin HC; *Hycomine Compound; Isoclor Capsules; *Kronofed-A; *Naldecon; *Nolamine; *Novafed A; **Novahistine products; *Ornade; Par-Decon; **PediaCare products; *Pediacof; *Protid; Pyrroxate; *Quelidrine; *Rhinolar products; **Ru-Tuss products; Ryna liquid; Sinarest; Sine-Off; Singlet; *Sinulin; Sinutab; Sudafed Plus products; **Teldrin; **Triaminic products; Triaminicin; **Triaminicol prducts; Tylenol Allergy Sinus Medication

Class/Type	*Generic Name:*	*Available in:*
CLASS THREE		
	Chlorpheniramine tannate	R-Tannate products; Rynatan products; Rynatuss products
	Dexbromphen-iramine maleate	Disophrol; Drixoral products; Sinutab Allergy Formula SA Tablets
	Dexchlorophen-iramine maleate	*Polaramine products
	Pheniramine maleate	Dristan Nasal Spray; Naphcon-A Eye Drops; Poly-Histine products; *Ru-Tuss with Hydrocodone; *Triaminic products
	Tripolidine hydrochloride	Actidil products; Actifed products; *Tripolidine
CLASS FOUR		
Piperazines	Hydroxyzine hydrochloride	Atarax products; Marax products
	Hydroxyzine pamoate	*Vistaril products
	Meclizine hydrochloride	*Antivert; **Bonine (used for vertigo, nausea, vomiting, and motion sickness)
	Phenindamine tartrate	*Nolahist; *Nolamine
CLASS FIVE		
Phenothiazines	Methdilazine hydrochloride	*Tacaryl Tablets
	Promethazine hydrochloride	*Phenergan products
	Trimeprazine tartrate	*Temaril
CLASS SIX		
Piperidines	Azatadine maleate	*Optimine; *Trinalin
	Cyproheptadine hydrochloride	*Periactin products
CLASS SEVEN		
Nonsedating antihistamines	Terfenadine	*Seldane; Seldane D
	Astemizole	*Hismanal

*Available by prescription only
**Available both over the counter and by prescription

H2 Antihistamine

The first H2 antihistamine, cimetidine (Tagamet), came on the market in the United States in 1982. Its primary use now is to treat stomach and duodenal ulcers. It is still used in the treatment of urticaria (hives) but has lost favor somewhat because it is a short-acting drug (frequent doses are necessary).

A newer H2 antihistamine, ranitidine hydrochloride (Zantac), lasts longer (two doses daily are usually recommended) and is less likely than Tagamet to affect the metabolism of other medicines that a person might be taking, such as theophylline or antidepressants.

Two other H2 antihistamines, famotidine (Pepcid) and nizatidine (Axid), complete the family for the time being.

All are used in treating stomach disorders, such as ulcers and reflux of stomach contents into the esophagus, which can trigger asthma in some people (see chapter 9).

Side effects of these drugs do not occur commonly. They include headache and confusion, and, even less commonly, constipation, liver dysfunction, blood disorders, rashes, and loss of interest in sex.

One new finding is that H2 antihistamines may have the effect of increasing the rate at which alcohol is absorbed into the bloodstream from the stomach. So be careful if you are drinking, especially on an empty stomach.

Tagamet affects the metabolizing of drugs and other chemical substances by the liver. If you are taking other medicines or are likely to be exposed to high concentrations of chemicals, such as pesticides, consult with your doctor if Tagamet has been prescribed for you.

Antihistamine and Decongestant Treatment

Many people manage allergy symptoms on their own, buying antihistamines and decongestants over the counter. In terms of cost-effectiveness as well as therapeutic effectiveness, self-treatment is a reasonable approach for short-term flare-ups of allergy symptoms.

The types of allergy that respond to antihistamine treatment alone, or antihistamine plus a decongestant, include mild reactions affecting the eyes, nose, and sinuses and some rashes caused by contact with substances to which one is allergic.

Antihistamines are not generally helpful with food allergies or with asthmatic reactions. Asthma attacks, for example, require a combination of treatments prescribed by a knowledgeable physician, typically an allergist or pulmonary specialist. The traditional antihistamines, the kind you can go out and buy yourself, are not going to help if you have asthma. (See chapter 9.)

Most allergists do not recommend trying to treat chronic allergic disease with over-the-counter remedies or sometimes even with prescription antihistamines. By *chronic*, we mean a condition that requires you to use antihistamines for more than three months of the year, in total.

One reason for caution here is that prolonged use of over-the-counter medication may mask the development of complications involving the sinuses, ears, or eyes. If you experience facial pain, pain above the teeth, ear pain or dizziness, or any vision problems, have your condition checked by a physician.

Even if no complications appear, if you suffer from symptoms most of the time, there are drugs other than antihistamines that might be considered. The possible benefits of trying to reduce your exposure to allergens, and of immunotherapy, or desensitization, should be assessed.

In selecting an over-the-counter antihistamine for short-term use, we recommend starting with the least soporific drug available. People's reactions to different types of antihistamine vary, so you may have to experiment to find a type that works well for you. Or you might prefer to ask a physician, not necessarily an allergist, for a prescription for Seldane or Hismanal, the nonsoporific antihistamines.

Buy the generic version of the over-the-counter brand whenever possible. There is no therapeutic difference, and generics are generally cheaper. Be aware that prolonged use of one class of antihistamine may result in a tolerance.

If you are giving a child antihistamines for allergy symptoms, keep in mind that children often react to drugs very differently than adults do. So do older people. It is best to consult with a pediatrician or allergist when considering any medication for a child or an adult over age 60, especially if the medicine is to be taken for more than a couple of days. (See chapter 16.)

Decongestants

With many kinds of allergy reactions, the patient feels a strong need for a decongestant: the sinuses are swollen, the nose is running, and so on. And there are many decongestant medicines, in both oral forms and topical sprays, available in most supermarkets and drugstores. Yet these drugs may be tricky to use. Some have a minimal or delayed effect. Some have unwelcome side effects.

Decongestants are stimulants that work by constricting the blood vessels. They are related to epinephrine (Adrenalin) and have similar side effects. Elevated blood pressure is one possible side effect. Others to watch out for are jumpiness, rapid heartbeat, and headaches.

Both oral and topical decongestants should be used with particular caution by people with hypertension, diabetes, heart disease, or thyroid disease and by people who are taking certain antidepressants.

Decongestants tend to counteract the sleepiness caused by antihistamines, so the two theoretically are a good team. But there are different schools of thought on whether it is a good idea to use products that combine drugs, as many over-the-counter preparations do. If you buy individually only the medicines that you are sure you need, say an antihistamine and a decongestant, you can adjust the doses to treat your symptoms precisely. On the other hand, the combined formulas are convenient to use and often effective.

Whether to buy medicines individually or in combination is basically a matter of personal preference. Just be sure to read the label so that you know what you are getting and what side effects to expect. If you are taking other medicines of any sort, ask your physician or pharmacist if there is a possibility of a problem arising as a result of taking the new medicine. For example, if you are taking an anti-inflammatory containing ibuprofen (Motrin, Nuprin, etc.) or any other so-called nonsteroidal anti-inflammatory drug, you might want to avoid a cold or allergy product that includes aspirin. Together, ibuprofen and aspirin can create quite a case of heartburn and possibly more serious gastrointestinal problems, including bleeding or even ulcers.

In the table we list some of the more commonly used pure decongestants.

TABLE 5.2   DECONGESTANTS

Generic Name	Brand Name	Comments
ORAL DECONGESTANTS		
Ephedrine sulfate	Generic only	Short-acting
Pseudoephedrine hydrochloride	Sudafed, *Novafed	Contained in many antihistamine preparations. A stimulant, with side effects that may include elevated blood pressure. Check with your doctor or pharmacist if you are also taking antidepressants or other medicines.
Pseudoephedrine sulfate	Afrin tablets	Similar to above
Phenylpropanolamine hydrochloride	Generic only	Fewer side effects than ephedrine
TOPICAL DECONGESTANTS		
For short-term use only—follow directions on label carefully.		
Phenylephrine hydrochloride	Neo-Synephrine	There are oral forms, but they may not be effective.
Propylhexedrine	Benzedrex	
Naphazoline hydrochloride	Privine	Longer duration of action
Oxymetazoline hydrochloride	Afrin, Neo-Synephrine 12 Hour, Dristan Long Action	Same as above
Tetrahydrozoline hydrochloride	*Tyzine, Collyrium Fresh, Murine Plus, Visine	Same as above
Xylometazoline hydrochloride	Otrivin	Same as above

*Available by prescription only

Decongestants taken topically, in nasal sprays and drops, are more effective than oral decongestants. They are very useful in treating the symptoms of a cold. But they are for short-term use only. It is very important to read the label and follow instructions. Topical decongestants cannot be taken for more than three to five days or more frequently than recommended without risking a rebound reaction, a more severe form of congestion (rhinitis medicamentosa).

Sometimes patients ask what medicine doctors themselves favor. No single product gets all the votes. Doctors' recommendations are based on a number of factors, including their familiarity with one product as opposed to another.

The basic similarity of many of the widely available antihistamines and decongestants is one of the reasons that the products are sold in such complicated combinations with such elaborate advertising.

Cromolyn Sodium

The drug cromolyn sodium, discovered in the 1960s, inhibits allergic reactions directly at the mast cell by reducing the release of histamine and other chemical mediators of allergic reactions. Moreover, it acts without the annoying side effects characteristic of antihistamines and decongestants.

The uses of cromolyn are not as wide as first hoped. The researcher who discovered it, Roger Altounyan, himself an asthmatic, showed that a person allergic to pollen, who suffered asthma as a result of the allergy, could inhale pollen safely after first inhaling cromolyn.

This discovery was a major step in the use of medication to treat allergy. It was hoped that the drug would alleviate a wide range of allergic and respiratory diseases. Experience has tempered early enthusiasm. As with most drugs, there are drawbacks and limits to the effective use of cromolyn. Nevertheless, it is a remarkable drug.

How Cromolyn Works

Cromolyn works by inhibiting a mast cell's output of histamine and other chemical mediators, even when the cell is in contact with an allergen-antibody duo that would ordinarily cause histamine release and the resulting unpleasant symptoms.

The full story on how cromolyn works is not yet entirely understood, but basically it interferes with the internal chemistry of a mast cell, depriving it of energy. It does this by inhibiting the production of enzymes that permit calcium to enter the cell. Without calcium, the cell does not function normally and does not release histamine.

Equally important, cromolyn reduces inflammation associated with allergy, and in asthma it blocks what is called the late-phase reaction, which can result in an ongoing tendency to asthma attacks even days and weeks after the initial asthma flare-up. (See chapter 9.)

Note that the drug is not helpful once an asthma attack is under way. It is a preventive treatment.

Because of the low incidence of side effects, cromolyn is worth a try in almost all situations. It is especially effective in cases of mild allergic asthma or in exercise-induced asthma. In the latter instance, cromolyn is more likely to be helpful for people aged between five and 35, but others can use it to good effect as well. There is no way to predict who will benefit from cromolyn, and there are patients in all age groups who successfully use this drug.

To work, cromolyn must be applied locally. For asthma, the drug is available under the brand name Intal, taken by means of an inhaler. For allergic rhinitis (hay fever), there is a nasal spray called Nasalcrom. And for allergic conjunctivitis, cromolyn comes in the form of eye drops that may help within days, sold under the name Opticrom. (With other eye conditions, positive results may be delayed up to six weeks [see chapter 11].) All three products require a prescription.

For asthma. A device called a Spinhaler was the original means of administering cromolyn in treating asthma, but the device is clumsy to use and requires more coordination than children and many adults possess. Today the most common means of taking the drug for asthma is with a metered-dose inhaler (MDI) or in a solution for use with a nebulizer, which creates a fine, misty spray to be inhaled.

One drawback of cromolyn is that it takes a while to have an effect. In asthma, often four to eight weeks of use is needed. Also, the effects are sometimes subtle, reducing rather than eliminating symptoms.

Exercise-induced asthma. For people who want to exercise but who tend to get asthma attacks after they exert themselves, cromolyn is often very helpful when used 15 minutes before exercise. Cromolyn is generally worth a try for children and young adults who want to play sports, because it has a good success rate with few side effects.

Very, very rarely a person may develop a sensitivity to cromolyn itself. If use of the drug seems to bring on asthma, stuffy nose, or other allergic reactions, it may be that you are one of those people who cannot take it. On the other hand, cromolyn is considered safe to use during pregnancy. Very little is absorbed into the body compared to antihistamines and other medicines that are taken orally.

For hay fever and other allergens. If you are interested in trying cromolyn for hay fever–type symptoms, it is best to get started well before pollen season. In perennial rhinitis, it may take several weeks before you feel a beneficial effect from cromolyn. If you put off seeing your doctor until symptoms have already developed, you may have to use the cromolyn along with some other form of treatment for a while.

Cromolyn is sometimes used to reduce symptoms from exposure to specific, known allergens. In other words, it's worth a try in the kind of situation in which you have an allergy to an animal and cannot avoid contact with the animal. But heavy exposure to allergens can overload the cromolyn mechanism, making it relatively ineffective. Cromolyn is good but not perfect.

Nasal Corticosteroid Spray Medications

Topical corticosteroid spray medications developed in the past ten years have become important in the treatment of seasonal and perennial (year-round) allergic rhinitis. They are available as beclomethasone dipropionate (Beconase, Beconase AQ, Vancenase, Vancenase AQ), flunisolide (Nasalide), and triamcinolone acetonide (Nasacort). The *AQ* means that the medication is in an aqueous base and may provide a slight moisturizing and soothing effect as well as the anti-inflammatory effect of the steroid.

These medications may take up to two weeks to work. They are best started before symptoms related to a known allergy season develop. They must be used regularly two to four times per day, depending on the drug and your doctor's recommendation. Nasacort may be effective if used only once daily.

The safety of these medications has been demonstrated in chronic use of up to seven years. Nasal ulcers can occur, but they are rare; therefore, a physician should examine the nasal lining periodically. Local side effects of headache, nasal congestion, and bleeding are also very rare. To reduce the chance of ulcer formation, the spray should be directed in different directions each time it is used. These sprays are also useful in the treatment of nasal polyps and in the prevention of their recurrence after surgery.

Anti-itch Topical Medicines

If you've ever had a bad case of poison ivy treated the old-fashioned way, you know why today people use corticosteroid creams and ointments. Poison ivy victims used to go around for weeks painted pink with calamine lotion, which actually did little to check the spread of the rash or to relieve the itch.

Treatment with corticosteroids is much more effective for eczema and for poison ivy and other types of contact dermatitis. These disorders (see chapter 12) can occur in mild or serious forms, and should not be taken too lightly. When in doubt as to the cause of a rash or when a rash continues to be troublesome over a week or more, it is best to see a doctor for diagnosis and treatment.

Poison Ivy Rash

A few patches of poison ivy rash, however, are not ordinarily cause to visit the doctor. Usually the rash can be diagnosed by anyone familiar with the effects of poison ivy and can be brought under control quickly with an over-the-counter corticosteroid cream. The same is true of an outbreak of dermatitis resulting from short-term exposure to something to which you are sensitive. The person who is allergic to chrysanthemums but includes them in the garden, the person who is sensitive to, say, flea shampoo for pets but uses it on the dog anyway—these people may develop itchy, burning rashes that need short-term treatment.

Strength and Usage Recommendation

Most drugstores carry low-potency corticosteroid creams on their shelves, and there are a couple of dozen stronger varieties available through prescription.

We've used the terms *ointment* and *cream* nontechnically, but there are distinctions among ointments, creams, lotions, and gels. Ointments are the most occlusive—that is, they block the penetration of air most effectively and allow the most absorption of the steroid into the skin. Creams, lotions, and gels are, in the order listed, increasingly less occlusive, and therefore more drying.

The occlusiveness of these preparations is increased if you wrap the treated area with an airtight dressing, such as plastic food wrap. The result is more impact per dose, but with some of the stronger preparations the dressing increases the risk of side effects, including skin thinning and infection. Never use such dressings without medical supervision.

As a rule, the fluorinated corticosteroid products are the most potent and must be used with the most care. (These products are identified in the table below.) They should not be used in sensitive areas, especially where the blood vessels are close to the surface—for example, the face, neck, or groin. Nor should they be spread over large areas or be used for prolonged periods of time. All topical steroids absorb through the skin. Therefore, if you are pregnant or even think you could be, do not use these medications without a physician's advice.

Side Effects

Normally, side effects are minimal. Local side effects may include itching, dryness, or loss of skin color. Contact dermatitis sometimes results from chemicals in the medications, especially the preservative Parabens. But there are several Parabens-free preparations, such as Halog, Lidex, Kenalog, and Aristocort.

TABLE 5.3   TOPICAL CORTICOSTEROID PREPARATIONS[a]

GROUP I (HIGH POTENCY)

0.05%	Betamethasone diproprionate[b]
0.1%	Amcinonide[b]
0.25%	Desoximetasone[b]
0.5%	Triamcinolone acetonide[b]
0.2%	Fluocinolone acetonide[b]
0.05%	Diflorasone diacetate[b]
0.1%	Halcinonide[b]
0.05%	Fluocinonide[b]
0.05%	Clobetasole propinate[b]

GROUP II (INTERMEDIATE POTENCY)

0.2%	Hydrocortisone valerate
0.025%	Betamethasone benzoate[b]
0.025%	Flurandrenolide[b]
0.05%	Desonide
0.025%	Halcinonide[b]
0.05%	Desoximetasone[b]
0.05%	Flurandrenolide[b]
0.1%	Triamcinolone acetonide[b]
0.025%	Fluocinolone acetonide[b]

GROUP III (LOW POTENCY)

0.1%	Fluocinolone acetonide[b]
0.025%	Fluorometholone[b]
0.025%	Triamcinolone acetonide[b]
0.1%	Clocortolone pivalate[b]
0.03%	Flumethasone pivalate[b]

GROUP IV (LOWEST POTENCY)

0.25–2.5%	Hydrocortisone
0.25%	Methylprednisolone acetate
0.04%	Dexamethasone[b]
0.1%	Dexamethasone[b]
1.0%	Methylprednisolone acetate
0.5%	Prednisolone
0.2%	Betamethasone[b]

[a]Grouped according to potency as determined by vasoconstrictor activity. Topical side effects are directly related to potency.
[b]Fluorinated corticosteroids
Source: Adapted from D. B. Robertson and H. I. Maibach, "Topical Corticosteroids," *International Journal of Dermatology* 21 (1982):59.

The over-the-counter preparations, being less potent, are unlikely to cause side effects. But do not use them on children under age two without checking with a pediatrician.

All rashes in babies should be medically evaluated.

Corticosteroids in other forms are invaluable in the treatment of asthma (see chapter 9).

There are also many other medicines helpful in the treatment of specific allergy complaints or in emergencies; these drugs are discussed in the appropriate chapters ahead. The medicines we've included here are primarily those that you might buy for yourself or might be prescribed for an allergic condition that is easily managed.

More serious or more intractable allergy problems may require a specialist's attention. If this is true in your case, then one of the approaches that may be recommended or at least explained is immunotherapy, popularly called allergy shots (see chapter 6).

6

Immunotherapy (Allergy Shots)

In 1988 *Consumer Reports* magazine ran an article titled "The Shot Doctors," which is what allergists are sometimes called, although not usually to their faces. The article maintained that too many doctors (not necessarily allergists) rake in money by giving allergy shots for years to patients who don't need them. Unfortunately, this is probably true. Nevertheless, allergy shots, more correctly called immunotherapy, have an important place in treatment. For those patients who respond favorably to them, they make life far more enjoyable.

How can you tell whether your symptoms will be diminished by allergy shots? How can you tell whether a doctor's recommendation of allergy shots is in your best interest, or only in your doctor's interest?

First, you want to be sure that you actually have an allergy and that it is the sort of allergy likely to be responsive to immunotherapy. Careful testing, plus a good history, can usually lead a specialist to diagnose an allergy—or the lack of one—correctly.

However, there are mail-order laboratories and shady physicians who are not particularly interested in the correct diagnosis. They want to persuade you that you have an allergy and need treatment, whether you do or not (see chapter 19).

Here are a few tips to help you avoid mistreatment:

1. Beware of diagnoses made exclusively on the basis of a blood test (without any physical examination or detailed history), especially a test other than the RAST.

Fraudulent or careless laboratories and doctors are apt to diagnose on the basis of a single test. As often as not, in cases of fraud or incompetence the result of the test is quite a surprise to the patient. This is especially true of food-allergy tests. You may be told that you have an allergy to beef or tuna or wheat or some other food that you eat frequently with no apparent harm. (This was the experience of a Consumers Union investigator who mailed samples of blood to several mail-order allergy-testing labs. Nonexistent allergies were detected, while his actual sensitivities were missed.)

2. Beware of diagnoses of unusual allergies (such as an allergy to the yeast *Candida albicans*).

3. Beware of findings of multiple food allergies to be treated by neutralization techniques and restricted diets. Food allergies do not respond to immunotherapy. (However, see p. 97 for a recent report from the National Jewish Center for Immunology and Respiratory Medicine in Denver.)

4. Beware of findings that contradict your own experience. A sound allergy diagnosis usually makes sense to the patient. For example, if you test out as very allergic to cats, your doctor would expect you to recall that exposure to cats makes you uncomfortable and a long vacation from cats makes you feel better. If that is definitely not true, the test result, even if genuinely positive, may not be relevant.

5. Before undertaking an expensive course of treatment, get a second opinion from a board-certified allergist. Even the best doctors will misdiagnose occasionally, and not every patient benefits from allergy shots. If allergy shots are working, the patient normally feels the benefit within a year, sometimes within six months. It is usually necessary to continue shots for a couple of years at least, but the idea is to continue only if the treatment is effective, not just in the hope that someday it may help. Fruitless treatment should not drag on for years.

Immunotherapy: How It Works

Frankly, medical researchers are not entirely sure how immunotherapy works, but they do have volumes of research findings that reveal some of the factors involved in successful immunotherapy.

In the late 19th and early 20th century, when immune reactions were first being investigated, scientists hoped that a wide range of diseases and toxic reactions could be controlled by building up immunities or tolerances in patients. By and large, this line of research has proved enormously beneficial, eliminating scourges such as smallpox and polio through vaccinations that create antibodies to the disease.

Nevertheless, the immune system is so complex that we are still doing basic research in many areas. In studying the immune-system disease AIDS, for example, investigators must search for a cure in many different directions, without knowing whether it is best to look for a vaccine against AIDS (which would be a type of immunotherapy), or to focus on inactivating the virus, or to take some other course.

Fairly early on, allergy reactions were distinguished from other immune-system reactions. Unfortunately, allergy was most obvious in its most dramatic form: an animal or human in whom the researcher was hoping to build an immunity would suddenly experience a violent, sometimes life-threatening (anaphylactic) reaction upon the second exposure to the substance.

Some of these extreme sensitivities can be reduced through repeated exposure to the allergen in minute quantities—in other words, through immunotherapy leading to desensitization.

In 1909, two English doctors, L. Noon and J. Freeman, began treating hay fever with pollen extract. Hay fever responds quite well to this kind of treatment. But the first scientific, controlled study of the effectiveness of immunotherapy in allergy treatment was not published until 1949. Since then, numerous studies have been done worldwide, and we have a much better picture (although not a complete picture) of the immunotherapy process.

When the body is exposed to a particular antigen (or allergen), it may produce antibodies to that substance. As you know, the basic allergy antibody is IgE. Overproduction of this IgE antibody is typical of allergy reactions. For example, in the season when ragweed pollinates, people who are sensitive to the pollen show elevated levels of ragweed-specific IgE. (It is not known why some people produce abnormal amounts of IgE in response to allergens and others do not, but this is an exciting area of research.)

Immunotherapy in allergy medicine is done by injecting the patient with small but gradually increasing doses of an allergen to which the patient has been found to be sensitive. When this is done correctly, the patient, instead of developing allergy symptoms, gradually becomes less sensitive to the allergen.

For reasons that are not yet fully understood, some allergens in very small doses promote production of a blocking antibody. This is an IgG antibody that interacts with the invading allergen, blocking it from linking up with the IgE allergy antibody found on mast cells and basophils.

A person sensitive to ragweed who is receiving allergy shots of ragweed-pollen extract shows elevated levels of IgG blocking antibody. During the ragweed season, that patient will not have the sharply elevated levels of IgE antibody that one would expect.

Researchers also have discovered that during immunotherapy there is increased production of suppressor T white blood cells. It is possible that these white blood cells inhibit the production of IgE.

Candidates for Immunotherapy

In trying to decide whether allergy shots are likely to help a patient, a careful doctor considers the nature of the allergy, its severity, and other relevant questions, such as whether the patient can successfully avoid the allergen or whether the patient is taking medication that might interact negatively with immunotherapy, such as beta blockers (drugs used to treat high blood pressure, angina, migraine headaches, and other conditions).

The age range in which immunotherapy is most likely to be successful is from five to about 40. Significant success also occurs from age 40 to 55. After age 55 allergy immunotherapy is less successful, although there are many examples of effective treatment in this age range. In all ages, treatment plans must be individualized.

Allergies That Usually Do Not Respond to Immunotherapy

• Food allergies do not respond to immunotherapy. (However, see p. 97 for a recent report from the National Jewish Center for Immunology and Respiratory Medicine in Denver.)

• Drug allergies are not usually treated by immunotherapy. But with certain drugs, desensitization is occasionally attempted when the patient urgently needs the drug.

• Allergies to feathers and kapok usually are not treatable by immunotherapy.

• Whether allergies to bacteria exist is a matter of debate, but in cases where they have been suspected, they have not responded to immunotherapy (that is, therapy with so-called bacterial vaccines).

• Cockroach allergy has yet to be shown clearly to improve as a result of immunotherapy. But new studies may tip the balance in the near future.

• Urticaria (hives) does not respond to immunotherapy. The same is generally true of eczema, except that eczema associated with allergic rhinitis or asthma may clear up following allergy shots for those disorders.

Allergic Rhinitis

Allergic rhinitis caused by one or more kinds of pollen produced seasonally by trees, weeds, and grasses (in other words, hay fever) responds to immunotherapy in 80–90 percent of cases.

Whether you would want to take shots for this sort of allergy might depend on how long the allergy season lasts for you. Six weeks of moderate sniffling might be bearable, especially with the help of nasal cromolyn, nasal steroids (as in nasal sprays), or antihistamines and decongestants. But if your symptoms last three months or more, or if they are very severe, then you might want to consider immunotherapy. This would be true also if, for whatever reason, you cannot tolerate or do not like the allergy medicines on the market.

Allergic rhinitis from molds may be a more persistent problem than hay fever, especially in humid climates, but immunotherapy for mold-spore sensitivity does not always work as well as one would hope. The available extracts of mold allergens are not as pure and effective as the pollen extracts. (This is because the mold extracts are made from the whole mold, although only the mold spores are allergenic.)

Many people suffer from perennial rhinitis caused by dust-mite allergy, which is then exacerbated by seasonal sensitivity to one or more pollens. This kind of rhinitis is a good choice for immunotherapy. Effective, pure dust-mite allergen extract is available for reducing sensitivity.

Some patients hope that by taking allergy shots they will be able to avoid the kind of changes in their home environment suggested in chapter 4. But unfortunately that isn't so. Both measures are usually necessary.

Animal Allergies

Sensitivity to animals can sometimes be lowered by immuno-therapy, but the better way is to avoid or reduce exposure to the animal (see chapter 4).

If avoidance is not possible—perhaps you are a veterinarian or you board pets for a living—immunotherapy is worth trying. Occasionally, even a severely cat-allergic person can be helped for a considerable time through desensitization. Recently, a very potent standardized cat-allergen extract has come on the market in the United States that seems to be more effective than extracts available so far.

Up to now, dog-allergen extracts have been less than optimal, but an improved product is said to be on its way.

There is little scientific data on the effectiveness of desensitization to horses, but many doctors report satisfactory results through immunotherapy. Sometimes the immunotherapy is enough if the patient also avoids grooming the horse or uses Seldane before riding. Be aware that an apparent horse allergy may really be a sensitivity to mold spores, which are common in stables, or even to pollen. The correct diagnosis, as always, is important.

Allergic Asthma

When there is an allergic component to asthma, especially if it is related to pollen or dust-mite allergy, the symptoms can be reduced by immunotherapy. The same approach as that used in cases of allergic rhinitis is appropriate: Diagnose the allergy. Limit exposure to the allergen. Desensitize the patient if possible.

A multicenter study on the use of newer, more potent allergen extracts in the treatment of asthma is currently under way in the United States. This study may provide evidence that use of these substances can block late-phase asthma reactions, which is a crucial step in controlling the disease. Some studies of the effects of mite-allergen immunotherapy have already demonstrated a decrease in late-phase reactions.

Incidentally, although patients with hay fever sometimes develop asthma, there is no evidence that treating the allergic rhinitis with immunotherapy can prevent the development of asthma.

Bees, Wasps, and Other Nasties

If you have had a severe allergic reaction (not merely local swelling) to the sting of a bee, wasp, or fire ant, it is very important, perhaps a matter of life and death, to get desensitization treatment. You should also learn how to use and always have available an EpiPen, which contains epinephrine (Adrenalin).

If you are stung, try to collect the carcass of the critter that got you or of one of its relatives (do not pick it up with your bare hands) and take it with you to your doctor for identification.

Allergy shots, when done properly, will usually provide complete protection against a single sting from an insect in the bee or wasp family. They also provide some protection against multiple stings. But any sensitive person who receives multiple stings should regard it as a potential emergency.

Allergy Shots: What They're Like

Allergy shots are typically started on a weekly schedule, although to speed up the process of desensitizing one can start by giving the shots twice a week or even more frequently.

Gradually increasing doses of allergen are given with each shot until a maintenance dose is reached. The maintenance dose is a predetermined amount or the maximum dose the patient can tolerate without a reaction—whichever comes first.

While working toward the maintenance dose, one must keep

to a regular schedule or else the dose must be held the same or reduced. For example, if you are getting a shot every week and miss two weeks, the dose should not be increased. If you go more than four weeks without a shot, the dose should be reduced.

Allergy shots are safe to continue during pregnancy, but it is best not to start treatment or to increase the dose at this time. The idea is to avoid a systemic reaction to the shot, which, although rare, could be harmful and possibly induce a miscarriage.

After the maximum dose has been reached (which usually takes six months to a year), the shots can be administered less frequently, gradually stretching out the interval to two, three, or even four weeks.

Shots are sometimes given seasonally, either during or preceding the season in which the patient reports having suffered allergy symptoms. This approach is not recommended. The best results come when the shots are given year-round. If you are being treated for an allergy to ragweed, the dose of ragweed allergen should not be increased during the ragweed pollination period. This applies to other pollens as well.

The shots are not painful. They are given under the skin (subcutaneously) but not into the muscle (intramuscularly). They are usually administered by a nurse, but a physician must be on hand in case you experience a systemic, anaphylactic reaction to the shots (with swelling of the throat, hives, difficulty breathing, and so on). If that happens, the doctor will immediately give you a shot of epinephrine (Adrenalin) and perhaps antihistamine. This will almost always take care of the problem. Very rarely, a patient may have to go to the hospital. There is an extremely slight risk that death may occur, but in the past 25 years very, very few deaths from immunotherapy have been reported in the United States.

The patient should be prepared for possible reactions. Sometimes the skin around the site of the shot becomes red, itchy, and swollen, forming a raised wheal. Sometimes the whole arm begins to swell.

Even if you have experienced only minimal reactions or no reaction, you must wait in the doctor's office for a half hour after each shot to be certain that you do not develop difficulty breathing or other symptoms of anaphylaxis. Most severe reactions occur in the first 30 minutes after the shot, so it is imperative that you remain in the doctor's office during this period.

Length of Treatment

Immunotherapy is often continued for three to seven years. Improvement should occur within a year of achieving maintenance. If this doesn't happen, it is wise to discontinue the shots.

There are certain circumstances under which a long period of treatment—a minimum of ten years—is advisable. In some cases, it may be best to continue indefinitely if the treatment results are excellent. This might be true, for example, in the case of someone with severe asthma who is much improved during immunotherapy.

Complicating conditions, such as nasal polyps or sinus or ear disease, may also dictate a prolonged course of treatment.

If it is difficult for you to get to your allergist's office, arrangements can sometimes be made to have the shots given by another doctor. Occasionally they can even be given in the home (although this is not recommended).

With home treatment, you must be scrupulous in following directions about refrigerating the allergen extract, measuring dosage carefully, and maintaining emergency medications.

Results and Costs

Allergy shots are expensive. It is difficult to come up with a cost estimate that is meaningful nationwide, because prices vary from place to place, but an average price in New York City for one allergy shot is about $40. A five-year course of desensitization will generally cost about $5,000.

The bills are covered at least in part by almost all types of medical insurance.

Among patients whose symptoms disappear or are reduced, and who then stop the treatment after, say, five to seven years, a lucky one-third find that the reduced sensitivity is a permanent condition. Another one-third experience the return of some symptoms but remain much improved. The unfortunate other third will return to their original allergic state. This tendency to relapse is very variable; relapse may occur within a few months of discontinuing immunotherapy, or even ten years later. Most relapses occur within three years of discontinuing immunotherapy.

Immunotherapy can be started again if your symptoms return, but it may not be successful the second time around.

There is no way of predicting which patients will do well on allergy shots and which will remain well if the treatment is stopped. But your odds of being helped by allergy shots are good, assuming that you are an appropriate candidate for such treatment.

Is the investment of time and money worth it for a treatment that may not yield permanent effects, even if successful? This is almost always a question that only the patient can answer. It very much depends on your circumstances. If you have limited medical insurance (perhaps hospitalization only) and are working your way through college, or working to send a child to college, allergy shots may be a luxury that you have to postpone. On the other hand, some patients can manage their symptoms with medication but opt for immunotherapy, which does away with the need for sprays and pills.

Although no doctor can honestly promise success in advance of treatment, all allergists have many happy stories to tell.

7

Food Allergies

Lucretius observed, "What is food to one is to another bitter poison." In ancient times a violent food allergy was a mysterious and alarming condition. Imagine a healthy guest at a Roman banquet suddenly choking and gasping, then collapsing and dying. It is easy to understand why many innocent survivors were suspected of poisoning the poor victims.

It is as true today as then that an ordinary food can kill a person who is sensitive to it. Today we recognize a variety of food allergies and, in theory at least, can distinguish them from toxic reactions. But even as recently as 20 years ago, food allergy was still a very difficult field in allergy medicine. The mechanisms were poorly understood, there were key gaps in our knowledge, and the entire subject was further obscured by a few physicians who developed pseudosciences about food allergy.

Recent discoveries have cleared up some of the confusion, although unfortunately there is still a lot more quackery surrounding food allergy than, say, allergic rhinitis. Also, food sensitivities are very complex. There are straightforward food allergies, delayed-response allergies (which are less well understood), and intolerances that resemble allergies but do not involve the allergy immunoglobulin IgE.

In 1986, the American Academy of Allergy and Immunology proposed definitions of various food-related allergies and sensitivities. The differences are not just semantic. Confusion over these terms has been associated with confused diagnoses and treatment.

Here follow the Academy's definitions (with the addition of a couple of subcategories):

• *Adverse reactions to a food or to food additives. Adverse reaction* is the global term and encompasses all untoward reactions to food. These include but are not restricted to allergic reactions. An example is "Chinese restaurant syndrome"—that is, the headache, tingly feeling, and other symptoms that some people develop when they ingest monosodium glutamate. This reaction is not a true allergy, as it happens, but those people who get quite sick from it should avoid monosodium glutamate.

• *Food allergy or hypersensitivity to a food.* This refers to a reaction, involving the immune system, to a given food or additive. The category includes common allergy reactions—for example, hives caused by eating shrimp. Most often the substance in food causing an allergic reaction is a protein.

• *Food anaphylaxis.* This is a severe, systemic reaction that sometimes can be fatal. It is a true allergy reaction involving the allergy immunoglobulin IgE. The symptoms, triggered by the release of histamine and other chemical mediators, include hives, swelling of the throat, a drop in blood pressure, wheezing, and abdominal cramping. Tree nuts, peanuts (which are legumes), and shellfish are among the most common culprits in food-induced anaphylaxis.

Note that there is a similar type of adverse reaction to food, called an anaphylactoid reaction. This resembles anaphylaxis, except that apparently the problem food causes release of histamine and other chemical mediators without IgE involvement. Strawberries may be an example of such a food. They can cause anaphylactic-type reactions, but no strawberry-specific IgE has been detected. Therefore, we call the reaction anaphylactoid, meaning that it resembles but is not an anaphylactic reaction.

• *Food intolerance.* This is the name given to an abnormal response to a food or food additive that is not mediated by the immune system. For example, people affected with lactose intolerance typically develop stomach cramps and diarrhea when they drink milk. The intolerance results from absence of the enzyme lactase, which assists in digesting lactose. The condition is common among older adults, especially blacks, Asians, Jews, and Mediterranean peoples.

Food intolerance includes anaphylactoid reactions and the conditions listed below.

• *Food poisoning, or toxicity.* This is a reaction to bacteria (such as the salmonella bacterium often found in poultry), products of bacteria, or chemicals present in food. The symptoms can include diarrhea, nausea, and fever.

• *Pharmacologic reactions.* These are adverse reactions to some chemical in the food that acts as a drug. An example is insomnia resulting from ingesting too much caffeine. Histamine poisoning, discussed below, also can be included in this category.

• *Metabolic food disorders.* These involve an inability to metabolize a given food. One example is lactose intolerance, mentioned above. Another example is favism, an enzyme deficiency that affects millions of people worldwide. The lacking enzyme, glucose-6-phosphate dehydrogenase, helps to protect blood cells. The disease is provoked by eating fava beans or taking certain antibiotics or other drugs. The result is severe anemia. Symptoms include headache, nausea, fever, and jaundice. Favism tends to be hereditary, especially among southern Mediterranean peoples, including blacks and Italians.

• *Idiosyncratic food reactions.* These are adverse reactions suffered by some people that do not involve allergy mechanisms. Sulfite sensitivity is an example. Sulfite compounds, frequently used in food as preservatives, can provoke a range of allergylike reactions, including a rapid, severe asthma reaction in asthmatics, which is discussed below.

Questionable or Speculative Allergy Reactions

Many substances and additives have been suspected of causing adverse idiosyncratic reactions. In some cases, the evidence against the suspect substance is rather thin.

One of the more controversial foods is sugar. There have been numerous accounts of supposedly adverse allergic or idiosyncratic reactions to sweets, especially hyperactivity and irritability in children. But there was little if any scientific evidence of such a sugar sensitivity. Recently, however, researchers at Yale University found that some children who eat a hearty dose of sweets, especially on an empty stomach, show a sharp increase of adrenaline in the blood. This will indeed cause anxiety and irritability.

A link between sugar and adrenaline production helps to explain what happens at certain disastrous birthday parties for children. But luckily, adults do not seem to react this way. And the reaction is not an allergy. No treatment is needed other than not force-feeding sugar to children.

It is a good idea to reduce sugar in your diet, but be suspicious of any doctor who charges you for this advice. In general, there is not a great deal of evidence that food allergies cause behavior changes or mood changes, except in the straightforward sense that if you are not feeling physically well, you won't be at your best mentally or emotionally. Of course, there are complex links between nutrition and how well one feels and functions. But on the evidence available now, it is not clear that food allergies are the mechanism for such changes when they do occur.

The idea that there can be delayed allergy reactions to food is highly problematic. With a delayed reaction, symptoms may appear many hours or even a day after the food has been eaten, while in ordinary allergic reactions symptoms appear quickly, usually within an hour or so.

A few delayed allergy reactions have been demonstrated. An example is milk allergy in infants. But there are numerous cases of suspected delayed allergic reactions in which it is difficult to determine whether the suspect food is actually the cause of the problem and whether the reaction is an allergy or an intolerance of some sort.

A case in point would be a child who frequently eats corn cereal or cornbread in the morning and vomits or complains of nausea later in the day at school. It may not be clear whether there is a corn sensitivity present, although there are diagnostic procedures of considerable value.

Ultimately, if avoiding corn helps the child, it does not really matter whether technically it was a corn allergy that caused the nausea and vomiting. But many children have been placed on restrictive, not necessarily healthy, diets because their parents have come to believe without much evidence that their children suffer from a variety of delayed food allergies.

Incidentally, researchers theorize that in delayed reactions, the offending allergen may not be in the food itself, but rather may be a substance produced in the course of digestion or possibly by interaction with a medication that the patient is taking.

How Food Allergies Work

There is a tendency to think that food allergens cause stomach upset and diarrhea, whereas airborne allergens are responsible for respiratory symptoms. But, as we've mentioned, molecules of an allergenic substance can travel widely in the body and cause problems far from the original site of entry or impact. Gastrointestinal symptoms, such as nausea and diarrhea, are common in food allergies, especially in infants. But the skin is another common target area, where the allergy may appear as hives or eczema. Before the allergen even gets to the stomach, it may react with mast cells in the mucous tissues in the mouth or throat, causing symptoms such as swollen lips. The sinuses and respiratory tract may also be affected before or after the food allergen enters the stomach. Numerous organs are involved in systemic anaphylactic reactions.

Some people develop migraine headaches as a result of food sensitivities. The mechanism is not known, nor whether allergy plays a role. Caffeine or other chemical substances in chocolate, and amines in cheese, may cause headaches. (See chapter 19.)

Food presents a complicated challenge to the body's immune system, for among the hundreds of thousands of substances that may enter the system, the body must distinguish between nutrients, wastes, and poisons. Allergic reactions are a mistake by the immune system involving, usually, a certain class of chemicals—glycoproteins—within a fairly narrow band of molecular weight. Luckily, the body is not likely to develop an allergy to just any food, or we would face a much worse problem. As it is, there are certain types of food that we know are more apt than others to cause allergy reactions. Curiously, among these problematic foods are some that are very common in the normal diet. Indeed, it is not unusual to develop an allergy to frequently ingested foods.

The onset of one kind of allergic reaction can make you more susceptible to other reactions. For example, if you are sensitive to ragweed pollen and the ragweed pollen count is high, you may also become more than usually sensitive to a food allergen, such as watermelon.

Some people also develop anaphylactic reactions when they exercise after eating or when they exercise after eating certain specific foods. Celery and shellfish have been reported in this rare category of foods that are harmful in combination with vigorous exercise.

The treatment is not to exercise for several hours after eating. One patient, a young woman who was sensitive to the combination of celery consumption and exercise, was told to avoid exercising after consuming celery, of course, and, to be on the safe side, to avoid exercise after eating anything. But her physician also prescribed injectable epinephrine (EpiPen) for emergencies.

Who Has Food Allergies?

Some food allergies are linked to the atopic diseases: allergic rhinitis, atopic dermatitis (eczema), and asthma, which tend to occur together in patients with a family history of these diseases.

With certain patients suffering from one or more of the atopic diseases, food allergies definitely play a role. The younger the patient, the more likely that food is a causative agent. The likelihood that a food is provoking flare-ups of rhinitis, eczema, or the like is greater if the patient has had a sensitivity to the food from a young age.

In general, children are more apt to suffer from food allergies than adults, and pediatricians are usually well qualified to handle most early allergies, especially in infancy.

Many food allergies occurring before age three are outgrown. This is especially true of allergies to milk and eggs. Unfortunately, new allergies can arise as one grows older. The allergies associated with hives, angioedema (swelling), and sometimes anaphylaxis often appear in late childhood or young adulthood, but they can appear at any age.

Food allergies can even arise in old age, and they may well be misdiagnosed at that time because the general health picture is complex.

Problem Foods and Additives

Certain foods and additives are more likely than others to cause adverse reactions. But there are no hard and fast rules. You may thrive on one of the foods mentioned here and react badly to some normally innocent substance.

Up to 10 percent of infants and children develop allergies to one or more of the following foods: milk, eggs, wheat, peanuts, tree nuts, soy, fish, and shellfish. The allergies to milk and eggs usually disappear as the child grows up; the other allergies tend to persist for a lifetime. A sensitivity to peanuts is almost always a serious, potentially dangerous, occasionally life-threatening, lifelong problem.

Many infants and toddlers, approximately 25 percent, are intolerant of orange juice and other fruit foods, and may get diarrhea or develop a rash around the mouth. These symptoms do not suggest an allergy and are not usually cause for any concern, although you should notify your pediatrician of such symptoms. You can try a different fruit or dilute the juice.

The foods that most commonly cause allergic reactions in adults are peanuts, tree nuts, fish, shellfish (shrimp, lobster, crab, crayfish), and mollusks (oysters, clams, mussels, and scallops). Less common problems are celery and fruits such as apples, pears, melon, and kiwi. Of course almost any food is capable of causing an allergic reaction. If an older child or adult has a reaction to one of these foods, that sensitivity tends to persist.

Milk

Milk allergy can be manifested by asthma, eczema, rhinitis, and gastrointestinal distress, including bleeding, pneumonia, and even anaphylaxis. Obviously, every parent should be alert for signs of milk allergy (see chapter 16).

There are actually several different proteins in milk that may produce an allergic reaction. Most of these allergens are heat resistant, so scalding or boiling the milk will not help in most cases, but it may be worth a try.

People who must avoid milk because of allergies should be sure to get adequate calcium and vitamin D in their diets. Vitamin D helps in the absorption of calcium. Sometimes, though rarely, a milk-sensitive person can tolerate yogurt or certain cheeses, such as goat's cheese. A vitamin-mineral supplement is also helpful in maintaining adequate calcium intake. A pediatrician should routinely be certain that plenty of calcium and vitamin D are included in the formula or in vitamin drops if a child has milk allergies. An adult who eats a balanced diet ordinarily has nothing to worry about with respect to calcium, but a milk-allergic woman should consult with a physician on the best way to supplement calcium, especially after menopause.

Cow's milk is found in the following: processed milk products, such as powdered or evaporated milk; breads and pastries, except "kosher parve" or similar breads; butter and margarine, except margarine made with soybean oil; caramels; chocolates and other candies; cheese; cream sauces and soups; ice cream, sherbet, puddings; pastas; some luncheon meats and hot dogs; certain nondairy milk substitutes containing caseinate; pies with cream filling or made with butter; yogurt.

Egg

Egg allergy also can be quite dangerous in children. It is the white, not the yolk, that causes the problem, and raw white is more likely than cooked to provoke symptoms. But even cooked whites may be potent allergens, and an egg-sensitive person may even have to avoid the yolks, since they can be contaminated with whites. Egg-sensitive children are rarely allergic to chicken and other poultry.

Reactions can include hives and angioedema, flare-ups of atopic dermatitis, nausea, vomiting, and anaphylaxis.

Youngsters usually become more tolerant of egg whites as they get older, but this allergy may continue into adulthood, and very sensitive people may even have to avoid preparing foods with egg whites. Vaccines produced in eggs may also cause a strong reaction.

Nuts and Legumes

Soy or peanut allergies are fairly common in both children and adults. Both foods are legumes, and in both cases it is only the bean itself that can cause a reaction. The oil of the bean contains no protein and does no harm. However, only the commercial, well-hydrolyzed oil is safe. The tastier, gourmet cold-press method may leave some protein in the oil. Check with your physician as to which oil is safe for you.

Unfortunately, soy formulas are the best substitute for a milk formula for bottle-fed babies. If your infant does not seem to do better on soy, it may be that she or he has an allergy to that, too. Your pediatrician will recommend a substitute diet.

One of the most potent of all allergens is the protein in peanuts. As far as is known, it has been responsible for more food-allergy deaths than any other allergen. The sensitive person must scrupulously avoid raw and roasted peanuts and any form of cooked peanuts. One must constantly be alert to the possibility that peanuts may have been added to a recipe. For instance, a Brown University student died suddenly a few years ago after eating in a restaurant where the chili had been thickened with peanut butter.

A peanut-allergic person must always carry epinephrine (Adrenalin), wear a Medic Alert bracelet, and never hesitate to call for emergency transport to a hospital at the first experience of any symptom. (See chapter 13.)

A peanut-allergic person should beware of hydrolyzed vegetable protein (HVP) in European food products. Peanuts are sometimes used in Europe to produce this.

A person of any age who is allergic to peanuts may also be allergic to other legumes and even to honey (the bees may have fed upon legume blossoms). Watch out for peas, beans, acacia, black-eyed peas, chickpeas (garbanzos), lentils, licorice, senna, soybeans, and tragacanth.

Soybeans may be present in bread, cake, crackers, candy, cereals, ice cream, lecithin, margarine, infant formulas, processed meats and sausages, salad dressing, sauces, shortening (including Crisco), soups, soybean noodles and pasta (of course), and Chinese food.

Allergies to tree nuts are most commonly manifested by hives and anaphylaxis. Occasionally gastrointestinal complaints may occur.

Nuts are very difficult to avoid because they are used so widely. However, here are the worst offenders. There are six families, and cross-reactivity may occur within a family (in other words, if you are allergic to one kind of nut, you are likely to be allergic to its relatives): Family I—Brazil nuts; Family II—cashews and pistachios (related to the mango); Family III—macadamia nuts; Family IV—English and black walnuts, hickory nuts, and pecans; Family V (nuts and fruits of the plum group)—almonds, apricots, cherries, plums, nectarines, peaches; Family VI—filberts and hazelnuts.

Shellfish and Fish

If you are sensitive to one variety of fish or shellfish, beware of other foods in the same class. For example, if you are allergic to oysters, be careful with clams and scallops, but there is no reason to think that tuna will be a problem.

If you are allergic to one kind of bony fish, you may be allergic to other kinds or even to all bony fish. There is a common antigen in all of them. However, there is no reason to avoid shellfish, unless you are allergic to shellfish as well.

Fish allergen can cause atopic dermatitis, hives (urticaria), and angioedema. It is rarely associated with asthma, but a very fish-sensitive person may get an asthma reaction from the odor of fish cooking. Fish allergen's greatest danger is that it can cause anaphylaxis.

Incidentally, a fish-allergic person may have to be careful in using glues made from fish extract. Fish extract used as a fertilizer is also a problem. In fishing communities, fish allergen can be found in house dust.

Wheat

Wheat allergy is more common in childhood than among adults. It can cause atopic dermatitis, and sometimes asthma and urticaria. A sensitivity to the gluten in wheat and other grains is responsible for celiac disease.

People with wheat allergy must follow restricted diets, because wheat is so widely used. It is ordinarily found in bread, cookies, and other baked goods; many beverages, including beer and malted milk, breakfast food and cereals; canned baked beans;

chili; flour; pasta; meat products such as burgers, meat loaf, hot dogs, and sausage; and sauces, gravies, and soups.

Additives and Contaminants

Food additives can cause a variety of adverse reactions. Most are not allergens themselves, but they may exacerbate asthma or other allergic conditions. Sometimes a food such as milk may contain small amounts of a drug, such as penicillin, to which a person is allergic.

Yellow Dye #5

Several food dyes have come under scrutiny in recent years as health risks. Tartrazine (FD&C Yellow #5), a coal-tar derivative, has been linked to bronchospasm in asthmatics, and to hives and angioedema. The reaction seems to be nonallergic, in the sense of being non-IgE mediated. The sensitivity is associated in some cases with a sensitivity to aspirin and other nonsteroidal anti-inflammatories, including ibuprofen and indomethacin. About 15 percent of aspirin-sensitive asthmatics cannot tolerate tartrazine.

People who have asthma and are sensitive to aspirin should probably avoid tartrazine. The problem is that it is not always listed on food-product labels as an ingredient. It is now used less than in the past, but it may be present in flavored drinks, candies, sherbet, pudding, frosting, dry cereals, and even medicines. Any food product or medicine colored yellow or green may contain tartrazine.

Monosodium Glutamate

Monosodium glutamate, which is naturally present in some foods, such as Camembert cheese, is widely used as a flavor enhancer by cooks in restaurants and in commercially prepared food. MSG, routinely used in many Chinese restaurants, is famous for producing the "Chinese restaurant syndrome" that afflicts some people after eating Chinese food. The symptoms include headache and general aches and pains, chest tightness, sweating, and nausea. It will produce hives in some patients and sometimes provokes a flare-up of asthma, which can be delayed up to 12 hours.

As mentioned above, this is not an allergy. Indeed, everyone will experience at least some of these symptoms if they ingest a large amount of MSG. Particularly susceptible people should avoid the substance. (Unfortunately, food manufacturers often do not list monosodium glutamate specifically on labels.) Many Chinese restaurants will eliminate MSG if the customer so requests.

Sulfites

Sodium bisulfite and other sulfite compounds are effective, cheap, and tasteless food preservatives. Unfortunately, sulfites can cause a range of allergylike reactions, from rhinitis to anaphylaxis. Anyone who has ever suffered an unexplained episode of anaphylaxis should consult an allergist to determine whether sulfite sensitivity might be the cause.

Sulfites also can cause severe, even devastating asthma attacks in asthmatics.

The cause of these attacks was a mystery for many years, because such a wide range of food was involved and sometimes patients would react to a particular food and sometimes not. It took scientists quite a while to figure out that it was the preservative, not the food, that was causing the asthma attacks and other reactions.

Fresh vegetables caused trouble because they were often sprinkled with sulfites to keep them colorful and crisp (it is no longer legal in the United States to use sulfites in a salad bar). Patients also sometimes, but not always, reacted to beer, wine, pizza, and other foods.

Today the foods in which sulfites are most commonly found are dried fruits and vegetables; gelatin products; pickles; sausage; wine; vinegar; some fruit juices; cider; molasses; shellfish; beer; citrus drinks; prepared potatoes and potato chips; mushrooms; and guacamole.

Lesser Additives

The artificial sweetener aspartame is 700 times as sweet as sugar and has no caloric value. The substance is believed to be relatively safe, but there have been some reported cases of asthma and hives associated with ingesting it.

The following additives also have been implicated in adverse reactions, but less is known about them.

Benzoates, butylated hydroxytoluenes (BHT), and hydroxyanisole can occasionally cause hives. These substances are used as preservatives in ready-made foods, bread, milk, fats, oils, margarine, mayonnaise, soft drinks, and instant drinks. Sodium benzoate can exacerbate asthma, although this occurs only rarely.

Papain, present in meat tenderizer, has been implicated in cases of anaphylaxis.

Toxins

Various types of food poisoning result from toxins produced by bacteria and other organisms. Some types, especially botulism, can be fatal.

A number of toxic reactions resemble allergic reactions, and one, produced by a fish toxin, mimics allergy almost exactly because it is caused by histamine. But the histamine, rather than being released by the victim's own immune system, is produced instead by bacteria in the fish. The fish involved are of the scombroid family and include tuna, bonito, mackerel, swordfish, sailfish, marlin, sardines, anchovies, and herring. The poisoning can occur when the fish have been inadequately refrigerated. Symptoms occur 15 minutes after ingestion and last eight to 12 hours. Typically the patient suffers nausea and other gastrointestinal problems, as well as hives, headache, and flushing of the face.

An allergic reaction to fish usually involves one person, whereas a toxic reaction will involve everyone who eats the fish.

Diagnosis and Treatment

The diagnosis of possible food allergies is aimed at determining whether allergy or some other disorder is causing the troubling symptoms. The next step is to pinpoint the exact food or family of foods that is responsible. Many times patients themselves figure out which food caused the problem, but it is best to confirm an informal diagnosis.

For example, some children who seem intolerant of certain foods actually are suffering from stomach ulcers or a preulcerous condition. Many people, children and adults, contract moderately serious intestinal infections or infestations that cause gastrointestinal symptoms, fatigue, and apparent food intolerances. For example, there is a parasitic disease, giardiasis, caused by *Giardia,* a common parasite in drinking water. The parasites frequently are spread by beavers in rural water supplies, and they exist in city water sources as well. Day-care workers who have to change numerous diapers are often infected. The disease can also be spread by sexual contact. There is now a reliable test for giardiasis, and antibiotic treatment is effective.

The patient's history is important in trying to narrow the field of possibly allergenic foods. Your physician may well ask you to keep a written record and timetable of what food you have eaten at what times, and what symptoms you have experienced. You can save time by starting such a record yourself before consulting a doctor.

If a certain food or family of foods appears to be the culprit, then you may be asked to eliminate that food from the diet to see if the symptoms subside.

If no particular food stands out as suspect, then the patient may be put on an elimination diet. All common allergens are eliminated from the diet and then introduced one at a time to see if they provoke symptoms. Common nonallergenic foods are rice, bananas, applesauce, and lamb.

To test for sensitivity to food additives, there is a liquid nutritional diet, available by prescription, that contains no additives. The patient may be asked to limit food intake to this liquid for several days to see if the symptoms subside. This is not much fun for the patient.

Skin tests can be used in diagnosis. A negative test is reliable in ruling out a food allergy. But skin tests for food allergies yield a high percentage of false positives—that is, the patient has a positive reaction to the food during the skin test but really isn't allergic to it. Doctors who have a vested interest in persuading patients that they are highly allergic—and unfortunately there are such doctors—may rely excessively on skin testing. *A skin test alone should not be the basis for diagnosing food allergy.* If such a diagnosis is made, it may be prudent to seek a second opinion.

The RAST (a blood test; see p. 29) is slightly more expensive and may be slightly less sensitive to food allergies than skin testing. RAST nevertheless may be useful in many cases, for instance, if the patient's skin is already irritated by eczema, or if the patient seems to have suffered a severe reaction to the food in question.

A food challenge test, in which the patient actually ingests the suspect food in small, increasing amounts, can be quite conclusive. But this kind of test should be done only in a hospital or a well-equipped allergist's office in case a dangerous adverse systemic reaction is provoked. A challenge test is usually ill-advised for any food to which you have shown a systemic reaction in the past, although sometimes it is important to find out if there is still sensitivity, and then a challenge must be done.

The means of giving the test food vary, but one way is to use a gelatin capsule containing the food in powdered form. If no symptoms appear, the dose may be upped on subsequent tests.

Typically, the test is done in a single-blind or double-blind form. In the former, the patient does not know if a food or a placebo is being administered; in the latter, neither patient nor doctor knows.

Among the types of test not recommended are cytotoxic testing (a type of blood test discussed in chapter 19), sublingual testing (the food is put under one's tongue), and intradermal testing. *The American Academy of Allergy has determined that cytotoxic and sublingual tests are not effective. Intradermal tests, as already mentioned, are risky.*

Treatment

Treatment, alas, is avoidance. For certain food allergies, your doctor may prescribe injectable epinephrine (Adrenalin) or antihistamines to keep on hand to reduce symptoms if you should inadvertently ingest any of the allergenic food. Anyone who has experienced an anaphylactic reaction should have Adrenalin always available. It buys time to get to an emergency room. (See chapter 13.)

The National Jewish Center for Immunology and Respiratory Medicine in Denver has prepared a report about successful desensitization to peanuts in patients with a life history of allergic reaction to them. This finding is promising if it can be applied to allergies to other foods as well.

As mentioned above, if you are allergic to a food you may be allergic to others in a related food group. A list of related food groups is provided in the appendix.

8

Drug Allergies

In 1900, the official U.S. government pharmacopeia, which lists all existing drugs, was a skinny little book of a dozen pages covering a hundred drugs.

Today, *The Complete Drug Reference,* compiled by the United States Pharmacopeial Convention, Inc., a nonprofit organization that sets standards of strength, quality, purchasing, and labeling for medical products in the United States, lists over 5,500 prescription and over-the-counter drugs. An adult patient receives an average of eight to ten drugs during a hospital stay. Seventy-five million adults take two or more drugs per day on a regular basis. More than 15 million Americans take aspirin regularly.

Thanks in part to these many medicines, we are now able to overcome most of the diseases that afflicted humankind and our domestic animals for most of our history. We live longer, and daily life is more comfortable with the relief of normal aches and pains. But for every step of progress, there is a price.

One price is that many important drugs can cause troublesome, even dangerous, allergic reactions in some people. These sensitive people form only a small percentage of the total population, probably about 5 percent. The chance of any given individual having an allergic reaction to a drug is only about 1 percent to 3 percent, because even if you are among the 5 percent that may develop a sensitivity, certain drugs are much less likely than others to trigger it.

Drug allergies, thus, are infrequent. But like food allergies, they can be quite severe, even fatal, when they do occur. The most notorious allergen among drugs is penicillin, which accounts for about 75 percent of deaths from anaphylaxis in the United States. Ironically, penicillin is also the greatest lifesaver of the past 50 years.

Many other drugs, especially other antibiotics, are occasionally allergenic.

Adverse Reactions

Drugs, like foods, can cause various kinds of adverse reactions: allergies, intolerances, toxic reactions, and so on. An adverse reaction to a drug is any untoward reaction or nontherapeutic effect of that drug.

Technically, the broad category of adverse reactions includes effects of an overdose. Side effects, too, are numbered among adverse reactions; they are not as universal and predictable as overdose effects, but they tend to affect significant numbers of those who take any given drug. Many antihistamines, for example, have the side effect of making most people drowsy. Theophylline, often used to treat asthma, may make your heart race. Antibiotics often cause diarrhea.

A side effect that is categorized as common may appear almost invariably or may affect only 1 in 20 people. A side effect that is rare may affect 1 in 10,000, or occur with even less frequency than that.

A drug intolerance is an exaggerated response to a drug. For example, people who are extremely sensitive to aspirin may get a ringing in the ears and feel nauseated after taking just one tablet. The average person would experience these unpleasant effects only after taking many aspirin.

There are also so-called idiosyncratic reactions to drugs. These vary according to the individual, and often are not well understood. It is believed that in some cases enzyme deficiencies may be involved. (An example of an idiosyncratic reaction is the bone marrow failure that occurs, rarely, after use of chloramphenicol, an antibiotic. This occurs in approximately 1 in 30,000 uses.)

Finally, of course, there are allergic reactions to drugs.

About 15 percent of patients treated with drugs experience adverse reactions, and very often these people wrongly say that they are "allergic" to the drug that caused the problem. But as we mentioned, only a fraction of such adverse reactions are due to allergy.

It is important to know the difference between an allergy and intolerance, because if you mistakenly report having an allergy to a drug, a doctor may be forced to give you a less effective medication to avoid setting off an allergic reaction.

Often patients think that if a drug gives them diarrhea, they are allergic to it. But diarrhea is a common side effect of antibiotics and other drugs, caused by changes in the bacterial environment in the intestines.

On the other hand, if you are truly allergic to a drug, the doctor must know this, because that drug or another in its family could cause you life-threatening difficulty.

True Drug Allergies

The key to identifying a drug allergy is that it resembles other kinds of allergy. For instance, you will not get an allergic reaction the first time you take that drug. A sensitivity must build up. But that buildup can occur quickly, with the result that allergy symptoms can appear during the initial course of therapy, even though everything went well for the first couple of doses. Moreover, some people are exposed to drugs inadvertently or without realizing it because some drugs are present in food we eat. A baby may be exposed to penicillin through breast milk. Penicillin and other drugs may also be present in cow's milk or in meat from farm animals. (One is not supposed to milk or slaughter an animal being treated with penicillin, but it happens anyway.) In these cases, someone will have built up a sensitivity to the drug without realizing it.

Assuming a normal exposure to drugs, drug allergies often appear in early adulthood, but there are no age limits. Some children have allergic reactions to drugs. Some elderly people develop drug allergies even after having taken a drug many times.

Occurrence

Frequently, an allergic reaction to a drug occurs within minutes to one hour after taking the drug. If you are very allergic, even a minuscule dose will produce symptoms. There are also delayed reactions that take hours to two to three days to appear. Rarely, there are reactions that are even more delayed. For example, hives resulting from a sensitivity to ampicillin can occur several weeks after taking the drug and last up to four months.

As a rule, the more rapidly the symptoms appear, the more dangerous the reaction. Symptoms arising within an hour of taking the drug are potentially life-threatening. The delayed symptoms are normally less serious, but still require evaluation by a physician.

Major Adverse Reactions to Drugs

A drug reaction in the first hour or first few minutes after exposure that includes the following symptoms requires immediate, expert medical attention: swelling (sometimes with hives); difficulty breathing or swallowing; vomiting or stomach cramps; itching; choking; weakness; and a sense of impending doom. These are signs of a dangerous reaction—anaphylaxis. Choking and difficulty breathing are caused by swelling in the throat that is closing off the windpipe. This sounds serious, and it is. That sense of impending doom is appropriate. You might die.

If you experience any swelling of the lips, tongue, eyes, fingers, or hands—even without choking or wheezing—call your doctor or an ambulance immediately. Do not take the next dose of the drug.

Typical symptoms of a drug allergy are itching associated with hives or a rash, angioedema (swelling), and sometimes a fever.

Itching is so characteristic of drug allergy that there is a medical adage: "Without itching, doubt drug allergy." The itching is often related to hives, which is the next most common manifestation of drug allergy.

If you are taking a drug and develop hives or itching, do not take another dose. Contact your doctor within the day. Your doctor will have to assess whether to try to continue the drug or use another.

Another occasional sign of an allergy reaction is a cyanotic, or bluish, tinge to the skin; in dark-skinned people, this can be seen in the lips, nailbeds, palms of the hands, and soles of the feet. and soles of the feet.

Joint aches and fever may also occur. If you develop rash or any of the symptoms mentioned above, report this promptly to your doctor.

Incidentally, one sign of drug allergy is that the symptoms usually clear up or begin to improve within several days after the drug is discontinued.

Of the drug-induced adverse reactions described in the discussion that follows, some are allergic in nature or include at least some involvement of the immunological system. Others exacerbate allergic conditions or can be confused with allergy.

Hives and Rashes

Acute hives can be a sign of a dangerous drug allergy and should be treated as a medical emergency, especially following an injection of a drug.

A sensitivity to nonsteroidal anti-inflammatory drugs may cause hives and in some cases be associated with chronic hives, as well as with asthma attacks (see the section below on respiratory manifestations). This sensitivity is sometimes linked to a sensitivity to the food additive tartrazine, a yellow dye. Unfortunately, the anti-inflammatories involved include some of the most widely used medicines for aches and pains: aspirin and ibuprofen. If you are sensitive to these medicines, your doctor may recommend a substitute, such as choline magnesium trisalicylate (Trilisate).

Rashes are a frequent manifestation of drug allergy. Commonly they are morbilliform, that is, they resemble a measles rash, with multiple tiny red dots all over the body. The rash is itchy but not severely so.

A morbilliform rash can be the result of a drug allergy or of a number of viral diseases. There is a distinguishing sign between the two, however; an allergic rash may cover your body, but it will not affect your palms and soles. A viral rash usually does not spare the palms or soles.

Sometimes an allergic rash progresses to become thick and very red and itchy.

Occasionally, when it is difficult to determine whether a rash is caused by the illness being treated or by the drug used to treat the illness, diagnosis requires a biopsy of the rash.

Most rashes are relatively harmless, but they may develop into exfoliative dermatitis. This is a condition in which the rash spreads over the entire body and the skin begins to shed. This is similar to what happens as the result of a burn, and, as with burn victims, there is great danger of infection. Some patients afflicted with exfoliative dermatitis, chiefly among the elderly, do not survive.

Exfoliative dermatitis can also result as a complication of eczema (atopic dermatitis) or psoriasis.

Almost any drug can cause a rash, but the drugs that most commonly do so include sulfa drugs, ampicillin (which is especially associated with rashes as opposed to other allergic symptoms), synthetic penicillin (such as dicloxacillin sodium and methicillin sodium), erythromycin, penicillin, cephalosporins (which are chemical cousins of penicillin), and hydantoin.

Patients with mononucleosis have an amazing 9 in 10 chance of developing a measleslike rash from ampicillin. Certain leukemias also tend to make one susceptible to developing a rash when taking ampicillin. By and large this kind of allergy is not terribly serious, which is a small favor when one is so sick already.

The rashes that follow treatment with penicillin and the cephalosporins are notable for their longevity. They may last up to four months after treatment is stopped.

Photosensitivity

Photosensitivity reactions occur when a drug that is present in skin reacts with light. Usually the light must be sunlight, but artificial light is sometimes sufficient. Diagnosis is usually simplified by the fact that the reaction is limited to areas of skin exposed to light.

Photoallergic reactions resemble contact dermatitis but can recur months after the drug is stopped, if the skin is exposed to light. Among many drugs that can cause these reactions, the most commonly implicated are sulfa drugs and salicylamides (used in medicated soaps and acne medications).

Phototoxic reactions, which are not allergic in nature, may be caused by coal-tar derivatives, doxycycline (an antibiotic), and other substances. A phototoxic reaction may give rise to an exaggerated sunburnlike rash that can blister.

Skin reactions caused by drugs applied to the skin, or by handling drugs or chemicals, are discussed in the chapter on atopic dermatitis, chapter 12.

Serum Sickness

Serum sickness is caused most commonly by penicillin but also by many other types of drugs, including cephalosporins, sulfa drugs and other antibiotics, phenytoin (used for epilepsy), and propylthiouracil (used to treat hyperthyroid conditions). Serum sickness is so named because it was originally associated with vaccines made from animal serums.

Typically, when this reaction occurs on first exposure to a drug, it appears one to three weeks after starting the drug. If the person has taken the drug previously, an accelerated reaction may occur within several days. The symptoms include itching (from hives or a rash), swelling, fever, headache, fatigue, pain and swelling in joints, swollen lymph glands, nausea, and diarrhea.

These symptoms may be mild or severe and last several days to several weeks. Usually recovery is complete, but in rare cases there is permanent neurological damage or involvement of internal organs, including the heart, kidney, liver, pancreas, and adrenal glands.

Treatment includes stopping the offending drug and taking antihistamines and oral cortisone, depending on the severity of the symptoms.

Drug Fever

Most drugs are able to cause fever in susceptible persons. Certain anticancer drugs, for example, ordinarily result in fever. Also, the injection of a drug can cause local inflammation in the area where the shot was given, and the inflammation can cause a rise in temperature. But in some cases the fever is part of an allergic reaction.

Fever associated with allergy can be confusing to both physician and patient, especially when an antibiotic is being used to treat an infection that produces fever. If after five days of treatment the patient is free of fever and then the fever flares up, what is going on? Is the original infection recurring? Is there a new infection? Or is this drug fever?

If there are accompanying signs of allergy, such as a rash, the answer may be obvious. But sometimes such signs are missing. To reach a diagnosis, the physician should try to find out if there has been a history of drug allergy in the patient's past. One can also try stopping the drug, and if allergy is the cause of the problem, the fever will usually subside quickly.

The drugs most commonly implicated in drug fever are penicillin and the cephalosporins, sulfa drugs, certain drugs used to treat high blood pressure (typically, methyldopa), and procainamide and quinidine used to treat heart-rhythm irregularities.

It is important to identify and treat the cause of the fever because more serious manifestations may follow, including hepatitis (liver inflammation), vasculitis (inflammation of the blood vessels), and severe rashes.

Drug-induced Lupus

Lupus (systemic lupus erythematosus) is a disease in which the body makes antibodies against its own tissues. These antibodies (autoantibodies) can seriously damage the kidneys, brain, blood vessels, liver, and heart. Certain drugs can produce similar effects, causing the production of antibodies, although no underlying disease is present.

The most commonly implicated drugs are hydralazine (used to treat high blood pressure), procainamide (for heart-rhythm irregularities), and isoniazid (an antituberculosis drug). Other drugs that may cause lupus are methyldopa (for high blood pressure), phenytoin (for epilepsy), and even birth-control pills.

In drug-induced lupus, the patient is likely to develop fevers, joint pains, and rashes—and these may occur months to years after the patient has started to take the offending drug. Usually the symptoms fade rapidly when the drug is stopped, but the autoantibodies may remain in the body for years.

Vasculitis

Vasculitis, or inflammation of the blood vessels, caused by drugs is usually associated with rashes, as the blood vessels of the skin are involved. But often the vasculitis shows itself in black-and-blue marks, especially on the legs. Other parts of the body, including the kidneys and joints, can be involved. The drugs that most commonly cause allergic vasculitis are penicillin, sulfa drugs, hydantoin (used to treat seizures), and allopurinol (used for gout).

Respiratory Manifestations

Certain drugs can cause nasal congestion. Common culprits are reserpine and hydralazine (both used for high blood pressure) and iodides.

Asthma can be exacerbated by a number of drugs, especially aspirin and beta blockers, the latter even when applied topically, as in the case of eye drops for glaucoma.

About 1 in 10 asthma patients is sensitive to aspirin, ibuprofen (Motrin, Nuprin), indomethacin, and related nonsteroidal anti-inflammatory drugs. You may be able to substitute Trilisate. Acetaminophen (Tylenol) is not usually a problem.

In rare cases, the asthmatic with nasal polyps who takes aspirin or another nonsteroidal anti-inflammatory drug may experience a life-threatening asthma attack. This sensitivity is not a true allergy, but it can aggravate asthma. It is rather difficult to diagnose and does not show up with skin testing. (For more, see chapter 9, on asthma.)

As noted previously, people who are sensitive to the yellow dye tartrazine (FD&C #5) or to sulfites should read labels on over-the-counter medicines and question their pharmacists about prescription drugs. Sometimes these substances are used in medicinal preparations.

The lungs can be affected by reactions to drugs. Among the problem medications are penicillin, sulfa drugs, and even, although rarely, cromolyn, which is used to prevent asthma symptoms. In cases involving the lungs, patients develop a cough seven to ten days after starting the drug treatment. A chest X ray shows a picture that resembles that of pneumonia. The blood count reveals increased numbers of eosinophils, a type of white blood cell often involved in allergic reactions.

Nitrofurantoin, an antibiotic used to treat bladder infections, has a number of side effects to watch out for, including fever, chills, coughing, and chest pain. These symptoms appear in approximately 1 of 500 patients who take the drug, and they usually disappear one or two days after the treatment is stopped.

Methotrexate can cause similar problems. It is an anticancer drug; it is prescribed for some kinds of arthritis; recently it has been used as a steroid-sparing agent (to reduce the need for steroids) in severe asthma.

Coughing is a common side effect of a class of drugs called angiotensin-converting enzyme inhibitors (such as captopril), which are used to treat high blood pressure. Coughing resolves after the drug is stopped.

Blood, Liver, and Kidney Reactions

Allergic and toxic reactions to drugs can cause changes in the blood, including a reduction in platelets and a risk of abnormal bleeding; a decrease in the number of red blood cells (anemia); and a decrease in the number of white blood cells. These disorders are generally noticed only when a blood count is done, either routinely or because the patient is feeling sick.

An increase in eosinophils is often associated with allergy, and is discussed below under "Diagnosis and Treatment."

Because the liver metabolizes drugs, it may become involved in adverse drug reactions. The symptoms of liver damage are often subtle or nonexistent. They may include stomachaches, nausea, or yellowing of the skin (jaundice). But in blood testing one can run various tests for liver function. The drugs most often associated with liver damage include isoniazid (used for tuberculosis), certain antidepressants and other mood-altering drugs, birth-control pills, and some antibiotics.

The kidneys, because of their general excretory function, also may be affected by drugs in the bloodstream, including penicillin and the related cephalosporins, sulfa drugs, diuretics (water pills), hydantoin drugs (used for seizures), and nonsteroidal anti-inflammatory drugs.

Penicillin

As you may have gathered from the frequency with which penicillin has been mentioned here, it is the major villain in the story of adverse drug reactions. The first reported death from penicillin was in 1949, and today it causes some 400 to 800 deaths per year. Put another way, about 1 in every 10,000 doses of penicillin leads to anaphylaxis. About 1 in every 100,000 doses results in death.

The age group most at risk is adults 20 to 49 years old. The more seriously ill the patient, the greater the risk of a serious reaction. Penicillin makes no distinction between male and female or among ethnic groups; all are equally liable to become allergic.

Over a period of years, one may mature out of a penicillin allergy. If you have experienced only a rash, especially a delayed rash, the chances are that, if it were necessary, you could use penicillin again under a doctor's watchful care. If you have developed hives and other signs of an anaphylactic reaction, you may never be able to use penicillin. Future tests for penicillin sensitivity should probably be done only in the well-equipped allergist's office or hospital. Desensitization is even more tricky, although it can be attempted in critical cases.

Variants of penicillin taken orally, such as amoxicillin and ampicillin, almost always cause reactions in people sensitive to penicillin. The symptoms may be delayed days or even weeks.

Cephalosporins, which are chemically related to penicillin, contain allergenic factors similar to those in the penicillin molecule. But cephalosporins are not usually as potently allergenic as penicillin itself. The oral cephalosporins include Ceclor, Keflex, Ceftin, Suprax, and Velosef.

People who are truly allergic to penicillin have about a 5 percent to 16 percent chance of reacting to a cephalosporin. Typically, if penicillin causes a delayed, mild reaction, such as a rash, then it would be medically acceptable to try treating the patient with a cephalosporin in a case in which the drug is needed and there are no good alternatives. The best procedure is to give the first dose in the doctor's office a little at a time over several hours.

Anesthetics and Insulin

Painkillers and various anesthetics cause allergic and toxic reactions fairly frequently. Some opiates, for example, may cause direct histamine release. If you have ever developed a rash or any kind of adverse reaction to a painkiller, sedative, or anesthetic, you should report this to your doctor. Possibly you should avoid drugs of the same type that caused you a problem. Often another class of drugs can be substituted.

Symptoms such as weakness, changes in heartbeat, and fainting when local anesthetics are injected are not usually due to allergy but rather to the stress of the experience. But if there is doubt as to the cause, and you want to know if you are in any danger using local anesthetics, skin testing can indicate whether an allergy exists. If the skin tests are negative, then gradually increasing doses of the drug are injected to be certain that tolerance is good.

Recently discovered is the fact that anaphylaxis and other severe allergic reactions can occur during the administration of general anesthesia. This is manifested during surgery by a sudden calamitous drop in blood pressure and even cardiac arrest. Other allergic stigmata such as hives and rash are not always present. This type of reaction can be confused with many other nonallergic reactions during surgery. It is essential to establish when an allergic reaction has occurred because it will occur again and can be prevented by appropriate premedication. This is a very important point, and patients who have had this type of reaction during general anesthesia should discuss it with their own physicians.

Insulin allergy can be highly problematic to diabetic patients who need this substance to maintain health. There are various methods of coping, which should be reviewed with a physician specializing in diabetes.

Chymopapain and Streptokinase

Papain and chymopapain, derived from the papaya tree, are enzymes used in a variety of products from meat tenderizer to toothpaste. Chymopapain is useful in treating herniated disks. Unfortunately, it also causes anaphylaxis in about 1 of every 100 persons treated. It is believed that exposure to meat tenderizer and certain grass pollen may predispose people to react badly to chymopapain.

Typically, patients are tested for chymopapain sensitivity by both an in vitro (laboratory) blood test and a skin test before the chymopapain is injected into the disk, but these tests are not always reliable.

Streptokinase, another enzyme, dissolves blood clots and is used to treat circulatory-system disorders, such as heart attacks and phlebitis. Unfortunately, many people are allergic to it and develop anaphylaxis. Currently the possibility of using skin tests to diagnose this sensitivity is being studied.

X-ray Dyes

X-ray dyes, also called radiographic contrast media, are often used prior to certain CAT scans, myelograms, angiography, kidney X rays, and so on. The dye helps the radiologist see the organ being studied. But the intravenous injection results in allergylike reactions in 1 of 15 cases, in dangerous reactions in 1 of 50 cases, and in death in 1 in 40,000.

If you have ever had an allergylike reaction to an X-ray dye, this must be noted in your medical records. Be sure to mention the reaction to any doctor contemplating such diagnostic testing. There are new dyes to which you may be less sensitive but which are not used routinely because they are expensive. One of these newer dyes, however, should be used if you have had any previous reaction, no matter how mild, to X-ray contrast media.

Also, pretreatment with antihistamines and corticosteroids is very helpful in preventing or damping a reaction.

Severe reactions are less common when, as in a myelogram or barium enema, the dye is not injected into a vein. But recently a patient with asthma suffered an anaphylactoid reaction several minutes after a barium enema was begun, and was saved only by the quick action of an astute radiologist. Reactions such as these are currently being investigated by the FDA.

It was formerly thought that a history of shellfish allergy was a predictor of reactivity to these dyes, but this is not so. However, a history of hay fever or asthma does increase the risk slightly.

Prevention of Dangerous Drug Reactions

Other antibiotics and painkillers, too, may cause anaphylactic reactions. Chymopapain, as just discussed, can be dangerous.

The single most important thing that you can do to prevent an overwhelming anaphylactic drug reaction is to stay within reach of medical help for a half hour to 45 minutes after having an injection of a drug, especially penicillin.

Oral doses of a drug are much less likely to cause a severe reaction than injected doses. Delayed reactions are usually milder than those that arise in the first half hour or so. But this does not mean that you should ignore symptoms associated with an oral dose of medicine, whether they occur soon after the medicine is ingested or are delayed.

Anytime that you have taken a medicine and develop any swelling or itching, go directly to the nearest emergency room or doctor's office. If you start to feel worse en route, call 911 for emergency medical help.

If you have found that you have a drug allergy, it is important that you mention this to your doctor before trying a new medication. *It is wise to learn which other common drugs belong to the family of drugs to which you are allergic. You should avoid that whole family of drugs.*

When a doctor prescribes a new drug, always remind her or him of your allergy. Unfortunately a doctor may have forgotten your allergy or, worse, failed to have taken your earlier report seriously. Another prudent safeguard is to check with your pharmacist as to whether a prescribed drug is related to the drug or class of drug that previously caused you difficulty.

To avoid delayed but nevertheless serious manifestations of drug allergy, it is important to notice and remember any and all reactions that you may have had to a drug in the past. A remembered rash or fever that cleared up suddenly when you stopped taking the drug may be helpful in diagnosing a troublesome reaction in the present. Alert your doctor to any possible sensitivity before starting a course of treatment. Ask that the information be included in your medical records.

Diagnosis and Treatment of Drug Allergy

Diagnosis of drug allergy is often uncertain, and treatment is usually simple avoidance.

This avoidance, by the way, can also be helpful in the diagnosis. If the drug is withdrawn and the symptoms disappear relatively promptly, the chances are that the cause of the trouble was some sort of allergy.

Elevated levels of eosinophils in the blood, together with other signs of allergy, such as a rash, indicate that an allergic process is present. But an increased number of eosinophils by itself is rarely enough reason to diagnose drug allergy.

Skin tests for drug allergy are typically imprecise and sometimes dangerous. Nevertheless, they may be undertaken, always under a physician's supervision, when it is important to determine whether an allergy really is present. This situation arises most often in the case of patients who need treatment for certain infections, such as staph infections, or for a herniated disk, or for some other condition for which there is really only one drug of choice.

Skin testing for penicillin sensitivity, while risky, is of value in that it reveals the sensitivity in most (but not all) instances in which a sensitivity does exist. Skin testing is also fairly reliable for sensitivity to insulin, chymopapain, and local anesthetics.

RAST (a laboratory blood test) is not recommended for diagnosing drug allergy at present.

If a drug-sensitive patient must have the drug in question, a program of desensitization may be undertaken under controlled conditions (preferably in an intensive-care unit). Penicillin and insulin are the drugs for which desensitization is most often attempted, frequently with good results.

The treatment of symptoms of drug allergy is usually with antihistamines and corticosteroids, if necessary. Often just stopping the drug is sufficient.

9

Asthma

Asthma, one of our most common diseases, afflicts about 4 percent of the U.S. population, or about 10 million people. About 10 percent of Americans develop asthma symptoms at some point in their lives.

Simply described, asthma is *reversible* obstruction of the airways, caused by muscle spasm or blockage by mucus or both. The most characteristic (but not universal) symptom is wheezing, which is a musical sound like a faint whistle, produced usually while one is exhaling. Lack of breath, coughing, bringing up mucus, and a feeling of tightness in the chest are also common symptoms.

The airways of the lungs are similar to the branches on a tree—an upside-down tree. (See p. 115.) Air moves through the main trunk of the tree (the trachea, or windpipe) into two main branches (the left and right bronchi) to the lungs. The bronchi, which are relatively large tubes, subdivide into smaller and smaller branches. The smallest, the bronchioles, lead into clusters of tiny sacs in lungs, called alveoli. There are millions of alveoli, and it is here that air is exchanged with the blood. Oxygen enters the blood; carbon dioxide is removed and exhaled.

In a typical asthma reaction, lung muscle tissue surrounding the small breathing tubes tightens; mucus production in the cells lining the airways increases; and the bronchial walls swell and become inflamed. Sometimes the mucus forms small plugs that clog the airways and take the shape of the air passages. When these mucus plugs are coughed up, they resemble bits of string or rope, ranging in size from about the diameter of a piece of spaghetti to the diameter of a pencil.

With all this happening, normal airflow is reduced, which results in a feeling of dyspnea, or shortness of breath, and sometimes a feeling that one cannot breathe at all (the term *asthma* derives from a Greek word meaning "panting," or "breathlessness"). Asthma can flare up anytime of the day or night, and many asthmatics wake up in the early morning hours with difficulty breathing.

The mechanisms and physiology underlying an asthma reaction are not entirely understood, but studies indicate that in the person predisposed to asthma the mucous-membrane cells lining the lungs may not be as tightly packed as is normal, allowing allergens and other molecules to get below the membrane to where the mast cells are. The mast cells may then release chemical mediators, causing asthma symptoms.

Also, people with asthma have an inadequate supply of a chemical called CAMP (cyclic adenosine-3',5'-monophosphate). CAMP, which is found in the body's cells, works to prevent muscle constriction in the lungs; it also inhibits the tendency of mast cells to release histamine and other chemical mediators that produce inflammatory and allergic reactions, including mucus production.

A theory currently being developed holds that people prone to asthma are affected by a dysfunction of one part of the nervous system. In the autonomic nervous system (which governs our body organs) there are two opposing subsystems: the sympathetic and the parasympathetic systems. They have opposing actions and should balance one another. One slows the heart, one quickens it; one opens airways, one closes them; and so on.

In the sympathetic nervous system, there are so-called beta-adrenergic receptors, which respond to epinephrine (adrenaline) stimulation by relaxing the airways and by increasing CAMP levels in the lungs. It is believed that in an asthmatic these beta-adrenergic receptors may not function properly, allowing the contrary reaction of the parasympathetic nervous system—constriction of the airways—to take place unchecked, unopposed.

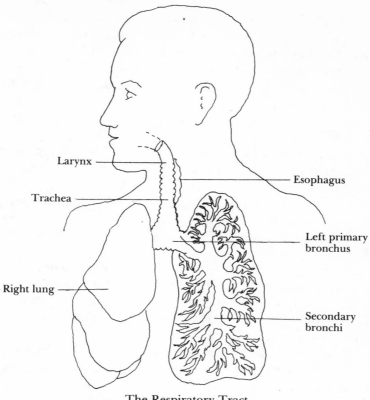

Larynx

Esophagus

Trachea

Left primary bronchus

Right lung

Secondary bronchi

The Respiratory Tract

Causes of Attack

Although this book focuses on asthma that is triggered by allergy, not all asthma is related to allergy. Asthma attacks can be brought on by exercise, cold air, aspirin or other nonsteroidal anti-inflammatory drugs, environmental pollutants, odors or irritants, smoking or exposure to cigarette smoke, infection, and laughing. It can also be related to gastroesophageal reflux, a fairly common problem, especially among older people. Acidic fluid from the stomach moves upward into the esophagus, which in some instances causes asthma to worsen.

One clue to diagnosing the kind of asthma resulting from gastroesophageal reflux is that the attacks come mostly at night and usually affect older people. When one is lying down, the stomach contents can more easily flow into the esophagus—gravity isn't helping to keep the fluid in the stomach. But another, even more common cause of nocturnal asthma is a natural reduction in pulmonary function. This occurs in all people at night and in the early morning but is exaggerated in asthmatics.

Exercise

In the past, many asthmatics were invalids from childhood on. Through advances in medication and a better understanding of the disease, most people with asthma can now lead full lives. In fact, they can lead highly athletic lives. Among the world-class sports stars who have asthma are the Olympic gold medalists Jackie Joyner-Kersee (in track) and Nancy Hogshead (in swimming).

Vigorous physical activity can improve lung function, reducing the impact of an asthmatic reaction. An aerobic exercise program can help asthmatics but should be undertaken in consultation with a doctor and should be done systematically, gradually building up aerobic capacity.

Most athletes with asthma need to keep inhalers with medication on hand, to be used as prescribed, usually before beginning to exercise. But youngsters will sometimes resist carrying an inhaler. It helps if the coach accepts asthma treatment as a matter of routine and if he or she treats the inhaler like any other piece of equipment. A physician or parent may have to explain to the coach that the youngster is physically fit.

Asthma on the Increase

Unfortunately, not all the news in the field of asthma treatment is good. In the past decade, the incidence of asthma and of asthma mortality increased, and we do not know why. The U.S. Centers for Disease Control reported that the incidence of asthma in this country rose from 6.8 million in 1980 to 9.6 million in 1987. Recent studies put the number at 10 million. The death rate increased by more than 30 percent, with total deaths rising from about 2,900 to 4,360.

There is some speculation that asthma medicines may have long-term adverse influences of which we are not aware. On the other hand, the very effectiveness of these medicines may lead some people to become overconfident and to delay seeking medical help for severe attacks.

Studies have shown that children, African-Americans, and the poor have been affected disproportionately. Blacks are twice as likely as whites to be hospitalized with asthma, and their mortality rates from asthma are twice as high. Rates are increasing relatively faster among young children. Urban areas account for an amazing 21 percent of asthma deaths in the United States among people aged between five and 34.

The concentration of asthma deaths in cities suggests that rising ozone levels in the air we breathe or other harmful pollutants (including sulphur dioxide and hydrocarbons) are taking their toll. Among the poor, lack of access to medical care is certainly a factor in the increased number of deaths.

Over the past 15 years, many dwellings and workplaces were sealed and insulated to save energy, with a corresponding rise in indoor contaminants and allergens. This may be exacerbating numerous respiratory ailments.

All in all, the picture is very unclear. For example, some studies demonstrate that on days with high levels of air pollution, hospitalizations for asthma increase and in general asthma symptoms get worse. But the findings are not all consistent, and in some instances other factors, such as viral infections, may be involved.

Asthma epidemics have occurred in Japan and New Orleans. In Japan air pollution seemed to be the cause, but in New Orleans the cause is believed to have been ambrosia pollen and mold spores.

In Australia, asthma mortality rates doubled from 1978 to 1988. In that country, a weed is taking some of the blame. *Parietaria judaica-pellitory*, also called sticky weed and pellitory, is a prolific pollen producer during much of the year. It has caused so much allergic rhinitis and asthma that the government has classified it as noxious, which means you have to destroy it if you find it growing on your property.

Stress

Stress is sometimes listed as one of the causes of asthma, but recent studies seem to show that although stress may aggravate asthma, it does not cause it.

In children, depression and asthma together seem to be a potentially lethal combination, although it is not clear exactly how the two are linked. A study of children who have died of asthma indicates that a distressed home life and depression put the children at greater risk.

Dr. Bruce Miller, a psychiatrist at the National Jewish Center for Immunology and Respiratory Medicine in Denver, suggested in interviews in 1989 that there may be an underlying physiological explanation for the role of stress. Stress at first stimulates the sympathetic nervous system (which would be helpful to asthmatics). But if the stress is not relieved—for example, if the stress is caused by the death or absence of a parent—this can lead to depression, in which the parasympathetic nervous system becomes dominant. As described on page 114, the parasympathetic nervous system tends to close the airways.

If this theory of the relationship between depression and asthma is correct, adults as well as children are more at risk if they suffer from both asthma and depression.

Late-phase Reaction

In several types of allergy, especially allergies to food and drugs, doctors are especially worried about the immediate reaction, which tends to be the most dangerous. In asthma, however, a delayed reaction, called the late-phase reaction, can be highly troublesome, even life-threatening.

The immediate, or early-phase, reaction in asthma begins within minutes of exposure to an allergen or other causative factor, peaks in about a half hour, and resolves within two hours. This reaction is caused by release of preformed chemical mediators, such as histamine and certain leukotrienes. These mediators dilate the blood vessels (from which fluid then leaks into the tissues); they cause smooth-muscle contraction (leading to bronchoconstriction) and attract inflammatory white blood cells. The early reaction responds well to Adrenalin-type drugs (also called beta 2 agonists—see under "Treatment," below).

The late-phase reaction begins about three to four hours after exposure to an allergen or other trigger and subsides in about a day. But it may leave the lungs in a condition of hypersensitivity, hyperreactivity, or irritability. The late-phase reaction is caused both by the chemical mediators released initially and by newly formed chemical mediators, which are created as part of the immune-system reaction. The newly formed mediators include other leukotrienes, prostaglandins, thromboxanes, and platelet activating factor. The effects of these substances include bronchoconstriction, inflammation, and excess mucus production.

The late-phase reaction does not respond well to Adrenalin-type drugs, and often treatment with steroids is required. Therefore, preventing or reducing late-phase reactions is vitally important in treating asthma. In asthma related to allergy, three types of treatment help to prevent late-phase reactions: cromolyn sodium medication, which reduces both the short-term and long-term inflammatory response in asthma; allergy shots, which reduce sensitivity to allergens; and use of corticosteroids, which also block the inflammatory response.

Diagnosis

The symptoms of asthma may be confused with ordinary bronchitis or a cold or hay fever. In the case of asthma that is caused by exercise, you may think that you are extremely out of shape. Unfortunately, the experience of an asthma attack during or following physical activity is likely to discourage further efforts toward physical conditioning.

Any of the following symptoms should prompt you to call a doctor:

- shortness of breath, whether following exercise, in the morning, in the middle of the night, or indeed at any time
- wheezing
- coughing up phlegm, especially if it is discolored or bloody
- persistent cough
- chest tightness or pain

In taking a medical history, the doctor should ask you about similar respiratory episodes in the past. Often patients report a history of frequent "bronchitis" when growing up.

Through a physical exam, chest X ray, and tests, the doctor will focus on determining whether the breathing difficulties are the result of asthma, heart disease, emphysema, lung tumor, cystic fibrosis (in young children), hypersensitivity pneumonitis (a dangerous, progressive condition affecting the lungs in some cases of untreated allergy), infection, or some other cause.

A disease sometimes associated with asthma is allergic bronchopulmonary aspergillosis, which can sometimes be detected by chest X ray or blood tests and often shows a fever accompanying the asthma attacks. This disease, caused by a fungus, requires a somewhat different approach to treatment.

In the physical examination, especially with children, one sees at times a distension of the chest resulting from asthma. The distension is caused by the asthmatic's reduced ability to exhale air from the lungs. The physician may also hear wheezing when listening to the chest. Examination of the nose may reveal nasal polyps or evidence of allergic rhinitis.

The pulmonary function test (see chapter 3) is often the key to making the diagnosis. The test will usually detect difficulty in exhaling air from the lungs. The diagnosis of asthma will become almost certain if the difficulty in exhaling is diminished after treatment with a bronchodilator (patients with emphysema are not helped much by a bronchodilator).

If the diagnosis is still unclear, a mecholyl challenge test may be recommended. This test involves inhaling increasing concentrations of methacholine while changes in pulmonary function are monitored. Below a certain concentration, the nonasthmatic will not show any reaction, but a person with asthma and certain other conditions, such as hay fever, will begin to wheeze and show a decrease in pulmonary function.

Allergens

If asthma is diagnosed, the next step is to determine what triggers the attacks. If the asthma is related to an allergy, this is often apparent in the patient's history and can be confirmed by skin tests or RAST (see chapter 3).

In children under age three, as compared with older children and adults, pollen allergy is less commonly the cause of asthma. In most of the country the pollen season is relatively short and sensitization is relatively slow to develop, so this form of allergy rarely appears in toddlers. But in places like Southern California, where the pollen season lasts up to eight months, asthma associated with pollen sensitivity can be a problem as early as age two.

Allergies triggered by nonseasonal factors, such as dust or mold in the home, can become a problem and lead to asthma at an early age, even among toddlers.

In patients aged five to 50, allergy of some sort often plays a significant role in causing their asthma. After age 50, allergy is less likely to be involved. But this is not a hard and fast rule. There are people who develop allergic asthma in their seventies, and there are young children whose asthma is not allergic.

The patient's history often reveals what is causing the asthma. Your doctor will ask if allergies run in your family. Are your asthma attacks more likely to occur in some places than others? At the office? At home? Are the attacks seasonal? Are they set off by odors or fumes? Exercise? Aspirin? Certain foods? And so on.

Sometimes the probable cause is fairly obvious. The patient reports spending a weekend at a house with a cat and getting an attack of asthma. Or the patient's asthma flares up after eating Chinese food, suggesting sensitivity to monosodium glutamate or sulfites.

In children under age three, food allergies tend to be as important as allergies to inhalants, such as dust-mite allergen, cat dander, mold spores, and pollen. From age three until adulthood, inhalants are much more likely culprits.

Food Allergies

When foods are associated with childhood asthma, the foods most often at fault are milk, wheat, corn, and eggs.

Among adults, foods are even less often the cause of asthma, but the possibility cannot be ignored. Sometimes the relationship between asthma and food allergy is difficult to pinpoint. For example, in one patient who seemed to have asthma all year round, no matter what she ate, food allergy did not seem a likely cause. But then the patient mentioned to her doctor that the only time of the year when she felt well was during the Jewish holiday of Passover—when she ate unleavened bread! The patient, it turned out, was sensitive to yeast.

A sensitivity to aspirin and other anti-inflammatories often causes problems for asthmatics. Another fairly common cause of asthma attacks among adults is a sensitivity to food additives, including FD&C Yellow #5 (tartrazine) and sulfites, used as coloring and preservatives in a wide range of foods, such as salad dressing, beer, cider, potato chips, and so on. (See chapter 7.)

Other Allergens

You should be aware that your asthma may be caused by some substance that you use in your work or hobby. There is a phenomenon called baker's asthma, caused by a sensitivity to flour. And one patient suffered weekly attacks of asthma, which she and her doctor finally realized always occurred a few hours after she had dried the family laundry. She was extremely sensitive to the fabric softener. The family settled for less-soft laundry, and the patient had no more attacks.

Some medications may make asthma worse, so your doctor should be aware, as always, of any medicine that you take at all frequently.

Aspergillus

Asthma can be seriously complicated by infection with the *Aspergillus* fungus. This common fungus is sometimes involved in baker's asthma, for example. It proliferates in unclean humidifying systems.

Aspergillus infections usually affect only patients already weakened—for example, those with abnormal immune systems or cancer. These infections are treated with fungicidal drugs. Allergic bronchopulmonary aspergillosis (ABPA) can turn moderate asthma into a fatal illness even in the absence of other serious problems.

Essentially, ABPA is an allergic reaction to *Aspergillus* fungi growing in the bronchial tubes. When this happens, the asthma patient suddenly begins to require more frequent doses of steroids to prevent breathing distress and begins to suffer from fever and at times coughs up brown plugs of mucus. A chest X ray is likely to show signs of pneumonia.

If a timely diagnosis is not made, the disease may progress to the point that the lungs become fibrotic (scarred). Steroids no longer relieve the asthmatic symptoms. The patient suffers chronic breathing problems similar to emphysema, and may eventually succumb to the disease.

Diagnosis is made on the basis of the clinical history of the disease; a positive result in skin testing for sensitivity to *Aspergillus fumigatus;* a high level of the allergy antibody, IgE, in the blood, as well as an elevated eosinophil count and the presence of antibodies to *Aspergillus.* Finally, a bronchogram or CAT scan may reveal a widening of portions of the air passages.

The treatment of ABPA is with a long period of steroid medication (prednisone). Immunotherapy is not recommended, because it sometimes makes the disease worse.

Avoidance of the *Aspergillus* mold is important. *Aspergillus* is most often found in crawl spaces and basements, especially those with dirt floors (it thrives in soil). Special attention must be given to humidifying and air-conditioning systems. An asthmatic who is being exposed to *Aspergillus* associated with flour or grain at work may have to change jobs. If you work in a building with an unclean climate-control system, you may have to look elsewhere for employment if management will not clean up the system.

Treatment

Often people postpone treating asthma, hoping it will go away. This is unwise. Although asthma may go into remission, over time, delaying treatment can be fatal.

Children with asthma have the greatest chance of getting better: 33 percent improve. Unfortunately, 33 percent get worse, and 33 percent remain the same. If asthma starts in early childhood and does not improve by adolescence, the person will probably have it for life.

Asthma that begins in adulthood usually continues indefinitely. An exception may be asthma that develops following a flu or pneumonia—sometimes this kind of asthma will recede in about a year.

In allergic asthma it is important to do all that one can to reduce exposure to any relevant allergens. (see chapter 4). But in some cases, immunotherapy (allergy shots) may also be recommended to decrease sensitivity to these allergens. Immunotherapy can be especially beneficial for people with allergic asthma who are inclined to suffer late-phase reactions, leaving them sick for days or weeks.

The decision to try immunotherapy is reasonable in the following situations:

- The asthma is seasonal but so severe that it requires significant medication, and skin tests or RASTs show a pollen sensitivity.
- The patient suffers from asthma all year, and tests show a sensitivity to one of the common perennial allergens, especially dust-mite allergen.
- The asthma is difficult to control with medication, or use of the medication doesn't fit with the patient's lifestyle.
- The asthma is caused by sensitivity to an animal, and the patient cannot (or will not) avoid the animal.
- The asthma is associated with rhinitis and the symptoms are difficult to control, with the patient feeling sick much of the time.

Adrenalin-type Drugs (Beta 2 Agonists, Sympathomimetic Drugs)

There are many drugs useful in the treatment of asthma, and among the most important are the sympathomimetic drugs or beta 2 agonists; they are in the Adrenalin-epinephrine drug family. They increase the production of CAMP in the body and are often the anchor of asthma therapy.

The term *beta agonist* refers to a substance that interacts with the beta-adrenergic receptors of the sympathetic nervous system. Therefore, beta agonists have a sympathomimetic effect, meaning that they imitate the effects of the sympathetic nervous system: they relax airways but also stimulate the heart.

Epinephrine (Adrenalin) is the strongest of these drugs. It is administered by injection in life-threatening emergencies, when the patient is suffering from allergic shock (anaphylaxis) or an acute asthma attack. It is available in inhaled form without a prescription (Primatene), but this over-the-counter drug is both less safe (because of side effects) and less effective than prescription inhalant medicines.

The prescription sympathomimetic drugs used routinely are often taken by means of inhalers. These drugs are frequently taken preventively, either before exposure to an asthma trigger (such as cold air or exercise) or on a regular basis several times a day. But a person with mild asthma can take them as needed, not exceeding the prescription dose. If they are needed more frequently, this is a sign that additional treatments with other medications may be needed.

Among the most widely prescribed drugs of this type are albuterol (Proventil, Ventolin), metaproterenol (Alupent, Metaprel), pirbuterol (Maxair), and terbutaline (Brethaire).

It is very important to use these drugs correctly. There are specific techniques to getting the right results from an inhaler or nebulizer (an electric pump propels air through a solution of the drug, and the vapor is inhaled through a mouthpiece). Pay close attention to your doctor's instructions. If the patient is a child, check from time to time to see if he or she is continuing to inhale the drug in the right way.

It is important not to use these drugs more frequently than recommended. Patients seem especially inclined to overuse inhalers. Excessive use is a sign that the asthma is out of control and that other medication is needed.

Side effects include shakiness in the limbs, heart palpitations, headaches, and rebound bronchospasm. These drugs must be used cautiously by people with heart disease, hyperthyroidism, or diabetes.

Cromolyn Sodium

In cases of mild asthma, cromolyn sodium may be all that is needed. It works best in younger patients but can be effective in all age groups. In somewhat more severe cases, it may be prescribed with a beta 2 agonist (sympathomimetic drug) used for breakthrough symptoms (see chapter 5).

Cromolyn sodium has a special place in the treatment of asthma, because it helps prevent the late-phase reaction, which can cause prolonged asthma symptoms. For chronic asthma control, cromolyn must build up in the body for quite a time to be

Allergies

effective. A trial of eight to 12 weeks may be needed to find out if the drug is helping or not. It can be used as a pretreatment before exercise (sometimes in conjunction with a beta 2 agonist) to prevent exercise-induced asthma.

Cromolyn is the drug of choice when it works and has minimal side effects.

Corticosteroids

Corticosteroids are invaluable in reducing symptoms in patients with chronic, moderate-to-severe asthma. The main corticosteroids are methylprednisone (Medrol) and prednisone. There are also corticosteroid sprays, including triamcinolone acetonide (Azmacort), flunisolide (AeroBid), and beclomethasone dipropionate (Vanceril and Beclovent). These have many fewer side effects.

Corticosteroids stimulate the production of CAMP, increase receptors for the sympathomimetic drugs so that they work better, stabilize the mast cells so that they do not release histamine and other chemical mediators of the allergic response, and decrease inflammation overall (including inflammation in the airways).

Corticosteroids can provide dramatic relief from asthma. Unfortunately, when taken orally they have a variety of serious side effects, including the suppression of the body's normal secretion of adrenal hormones, which are vital to the correct function of many organs of the body and to an effective physiological response to stress. They also cause fluid retention and sometimes weight gain, giving patients an undesirable moon-faced appearance. In long-term use one must watch out for osteoporosis (bone weakening), diabetes, high blood pressure, the development of cataracts and glaucoma, the development of stomach ulcers, and loss of potassium (signaled by a feeling of weakness, muscle cramping, and eventually heart arrhythmia).

Even the sprays have some side effects. Cough and hoarseness occur occasionally. The sprays may also sometimes cause a fungal infection of the throat, which can usually be prevented by rinsing the back of the mouth with water after using the spray or by using an extender device (Aerochamber, Inspir-ease) to deliver the medication more directly into the airways.

Naturally, given the side effects of oral corticosteroids, both patients and their doctors are usually eager to reduce or stop their use as soon as it is safe to do so. This may be possible when the asthma becomes stable, or perhaps through the use of other medication, such as inhaled corticosteroids. But the correct way to stop is slowly, through a weaning process.

If you are taking oral corticosteroids, do not try to discontinue use all at once. This can be dangerous, even fatal.

Your doctor should give you very detailed instructions on how to reduce your steroid dosages. In general, oral steroids are given every other day, when possible, to avoid entirely suppressing adrenal-gland function and causing other side effects.

If you are on high daily doses of oral corticosteroids, there are steroid-sparing drugs that may make it possible to taper off the basic steroid medication. These drugs include troleandomycin (TAO), which is an antibiotic; methotrexate, an anticancer drug that is also an anti-inflammatory; and oral gold, which is also an anti-inflammatory. But these drugs have certain toxicities and should be administered only by physicians experienced in their use.

If you are on regular doses of oral corticosteroids or high doses of inhaled steroids, or have been on either in the past year, you should wear a Medic Alert bracelet, because in an emergency or during surgery you may need additional corticosteroids to supplement your weakened adrenal glands. The suppression of the adrenal glands can last up to 18 months after you have stopped taking the drug.

Theophylline

A traditional asthma medication, prescribed in a wide range of forms and strengths, is theophylline. It is used now somewhat less than formerly but is still an important tool in asthma management.

Theophylline opens the bronchial passages. It may work in

part by interfering with the action of an enzyme (phosphodies-terase) that breaks down CAMP—that helpful chemical that counteracts bronchoconstriction. Asthmatics need more CAMP than they have, and they definitely do not need to have it broken down.

In some patients theophylline acts as a stimulant, interacting with numerous other drugs, so there should be good, regular communication between doctor and patient to make certain the drug is being used appropriately. It can be prescribed in a long-acting form or shorter-acting forms, depending on individual needs. For example, long-acting theophylline, when taken in the evening, sometimes helps to control nocturnal symptoms.

The purpose of theophylline is to prevent an asthma attack from taking place and to maintain good pulmonary function throughout the day. It must reach a certain level in the blood-stream to be effective. Ideally, this drug should be taken before an asthma attack is under way. The sufferer should usually take it on a constant basis, or throughout a period of time in which the asthma may flare up, such as after a viral infection.

A patient should not self-medicate with larger or smaller doses of the drug. Too much in a person's system can be dangerous, as can too little. The average range in which patients do better is 10 to 20 micrograms per milliliter of blood; over 20 is too high. A doctor should test blood levels of theophylline periodi-cally if the patient is being maintained on the drug, and espe-cially if the patient's condition changes.

The elimination of theophylline from one's system is slowed down by certain medications (erythromycin, cimetidine, and others), by high-carbohydrate, low-protein diets, and by diseases such as viral infections and liver and heart disease; even flu shots may have this effect. If you continue your regular doses of theo-phylline while it is being eliminated less effectively by your blood, levels of the drug will rise.

Conversely, high-protein, low-carbohydrate diets, charcoal-broiled meats, cigarette smoking, and certain medications like phenobarbital and phenytoin may cause theophylline levels to fall. When this happens, asthma that has been stabilized may get worse. Therefore, you and your doctor should maintain good communication about what is going on in your life to be sure that theophylline medication is achieving the blood levels that work best for you.

New Understanding of Asthma

Significant advances in the understanding of asthma as a disease of inflammation in the airways took place in the late 1980s. The trend in management has shifted toward earlier use of anti-inflammatory drugs—cromolyn and inhaled corticosteroids. In 1991, the National Heart, Lung and Blood Institute (a branch of the National Institutes of Health) issued guidelines incorporating these changes to all physicians in order to update their management of asthma. These advances are reflected in the sections below on the treatment of mild, moderate, and severe asthma. The most noticeable change is a shift from reliance on theophylline as a first-line drug, as was the case from the 1960s to the early 1980s, to inhaled beta 2 agonists and inhaled anti-inflammatory drugs such as cromolyn and corticosteroids. Looking ahead, there may be further changes in management as new drugs are introduced.

If you have asthma, select a doctor who is aware of new methods being introduced. A specialist associated with a teaching hospital usually will be up-to-date. Educating yourself by following medical news from a reliable source is also an important protection against continuing to be treated with outdated methods.

Self-monitoring

With asthma, it can sometimes be very difficult to figure out whether symptoms you are feeling are serious or not. Feelings of anxiety, rapid heartbeat, breathlessness, or nervousness can be due to lack of oxygen because of the asthma, or to the effects of certain medications, or to anxiety or to all three causes.

Acute Attacks

Asthma attacks vary from person to person and time to time. An acute attack can begin suddenly, peaking in minutes, or develop more gradually over hours or days. Death sometimes occurs because a patient does not realize how stressful prolonged respiratory difficulty can be for the functioning of the entire body.

The earlier you are aware that you may be in trouble, the

better you will be able to manage the attack. You should also have a plan worked out with your physician on how to handle emergencies and who will cover if the physician is not available. Your doctor may advise you to keep a peak-flow meter at home to test respiratory function yourself. A drop in peak flow may be a warning that an attack is approaching and that an adjustment in medication is needed.

You should know what medicines to take or increase in bad times, and should always be able to reach your doctor to discuss changes in medication and if a trip to an emergency room may be in order.

Signs that your asthma is getting worse include the following:

- You are using your inhaler more and more frequently.
- You are not getting the relief from your inhaler that you are used to getting.
- You awaken during the morning with more than usual tightness in your chest, or you awaken at night and have to use your inhaler, and this is not part of your ordinary routine.
- Everyday activities leave you feeling more winded or breathless than you would ordinarily expect.
- Your cough has increased and the sputum is more sticky or difficult to get up, or has changed color to yellow or green.

If you experience any of the above changes, do not wait until there is a crisis. Call your doctor.

Mild Asthma

In adults. If you as an adult have mild asthma, your symptoms occur no more than one to two times per week and you are relatively free of asthma symptoms between these episodes. You may have exercise-induced asthma and be awakened from sleep by asthma no more than a couple of times per month.

An inhaled beta 2 agonist such as albuterol (Proventil, Ventolin), metaproterenol (Alupent), pirbuterol (Maxair), or terbutaline (Brethaire) as a preventive bronchial dilator, or at the first signs of asthma, is adequate treatment. Cromolyn sodium inhaled before exposure to triggers such as cold air, exercise, or allergens may be used in addition to or substituted for the beta 2 agonist preventive treatment. If it is used as a substitute, you must also have a beta 2 agonist to treat any symptoms of asthma that occur, since cromolyn will not treat symptoms.

In children. Therapy for mild asthma in children is essentially the same as for adults—an inhaled beta 2 agonist taken as needed. Children over age five can usually use a metered-dose inhaler (MDI). Children age three to five can usually use one if a spacer is added. The preferred treatment is nebulized beta 2 agonist medication with perhaps an oral beta 2 agonist when the child less than three is away from the nebulizer (e.g., when not at home). A dry powder inhaled form of albuterol (Ventolin Rotocaps) may be considered, since the medication in this device is removed from the chamber by inhaling from it (breath-actuated), and less coordination is needed.

Moderate Asthma

In adults. You have moderate asthma if exacerbations of cough or wheeze occur more frequently than twice weekly. You also have symptoms in between these flare-ups. Your exercise tolerance is decreased, and nocturnal symptoms and awakening occur up to several times per week.

There are several treatment options. The preferred treatment is a beta 2 agonist used as needed up to three to four times daily, plus an anti-inflammatory agent such as inhaled cromolyn sodium or inhaled corticosteroids (AeroBid, Azmacort, Beclovent, or Vanceril). An alternative treatment would be the use of a long-acting theophylline preparation (e.g., Slo-Bid, Theo-Dur, or Uniphyl) with an inhaled beta 2 agonist as needed three to four times daily to treat breakthrough symptoms. If symptoms are not well controlled, options include increasing the number of puffs of the inhaled corticosteroid and/or adding an oral beta 2 agonist (Brethine, Proventil, or Ventolin).

Occasionally, short courses of treatment with "bursts" of oral corticosteroids (prednisone or methylprednisolone) may be needed to control more severe exacerbations, perhaps due to upper respiratory infections (colds) or severe allergic exposures.

To control frequent nocturnal awakening caused by asthma, a long-acting theophylline (Uniphyl) and/or long-acting oral beta 2 agonist (Proventil Repetabs) may be added at 8:00 P.M. or at bedtime, respectively.

In children. The definition of moderate asthma for children is similar to that of adults, but treatment differs a bit. The anti-inflammatory agent cromolyn should be tried first, and then if necessary an inhaled steroid should be added. This is because there is a longer experience with cromolyn and its safety is better documented in children, although this may change over time as the safety of inhaled steroids in children is more fully documented. Children who cannot use an MDI with a spacer (i.e., younger than three to four years old) will have to get cromolyn via a nebulizer. Nebulized steroids are not available (although some physicians are spraying MDI steroids into a nebulizer and aerosolizing them with success).

If the inhaled steroid is added and the asthma stabilizes after two to four weeks, the cromolyn may be stopped.

Severe Asthma

In adults. You have severe asthma if you wheeze daily and exacerbations are frequent and severe. You may have to visit an emergency room several times per year because of asthma attacks, and you may be hospitalized on occasion. Your symptoms are almost always present, and you can do very little exercise. You awaken almost nightly and experience chest tightness every morning.

Treatment of severe asthma involves the use of the anti-inflammatory agents mentioned, cromolyn and/or inhaled corticosteroids. The latter may be used in high doses. A long-acting theophylline may be added especially to control nocturnal symptoms that cause awakening. Oral beta 2 agonists may be added at bedtime, also to control nocturnal symptoms. A nebulizer may be recommended for delivery of the medication to control severe attacks.

Occasionally, oral corticosteroids may need to be added in a "burst" fashion—one week of a high daily dose, perhaps in divided doses, then tapered off over the next week. In more severe cases it may be necessary to take oral steroids on alternate days or even daily. In these situations of continuous use of oral steroids, attempts should be made to use the lowest possible dose. Other drugs—such as TAO, oral gold, or methotrexate—may be added to try to lower the steroid dosage in someone requiring it daily.

It is recommended that adults with severe asthma be evaluated by an asthma specialist. Certain patients with mild or moderate asthma may also benefit from this evaluation.

Also, the therapy for mild, moderate, and severe asthma must include patient education about preventing symptoms, including education about environmental control if allergens or irritants in the environment are important triggers of asthma. The patient must also be taught how to keep asthma under control.

In children. The definition of and treatment of severe asthma are essentially the same for children as for adults. Again, children less than three to four years old may not be able to use inhaled steroids, even with a spacer, although some physicians are spraying MDI steroids with some success into a nebulizer and aerosolizing them. Until the children reach the age when this is an option, oral steroids may be required frequently. This is unfortunate, since steroids can inhibit a child's growth.

It is recommended that children with severe asthma be evaluated by an asthma specialist. Certain patients with mild or moderate asthma may also benefit from this evaluation.

Also, the therapy for mild, moderate, and severe asthma must include patient (and parent) education about preventing symptoms, including education about environmental control if allergens or irritants in the environment are important triggers of asthma. The child must be taught ways to keep asthma under control.

Today, with proper medical attention, most asthma sufferers—even those with severe asthma—can lead full, productive lives.

10

Hay Fever and Other Forms of Rhinitis

Nature chooses adolescence, when most young people are acutely concerned about their physical appearance, to be unkind. This is the time acne appears. It is also when many teenagers develop the characteristic symptoms of allergic rhinitis—runny nose, itchy eyes, and a tendency to sneeze repeatedly. Indeed, teenagers are more prone than any other age group to develop rhinitis; about 30 percent of adolescents suffer from allergic and nonallergic rhinitis, compared with 10 percent of the total population.

At whatever age it first strikes, rhinitis can be seasonal or perennial, allergic or nonallergic in nature. As the name suggests, perennial allergic rhinitis is a year-round problem, caused by a sensitivity to dust-mite allergen, household molds, pets, or other allergens to which you may be exposed no matter the season. It is often aggravated by seasonal allergies.

Seasonal allergic rhinitis is caused by a sensitivity to the pollen of grasses, ragweed, or trees, and in some cases by a sensitivity to certain molds. It is popularly known as hay fever, although there is no fever and the disease usually has nothing to do with hay.

In the eastern United States, approximately 75 percent of seasonal rhinitis is associated with allergy to ragweed. A sensitivity to grass pollen affects about 50 percent of those with hay fever, and a sensitivity to tree pollen is present in about 10 percent.

The reason the figures add up to more than 100 percent is that sensitivities overlap, with a few people (about 5 percent to 10 percent) allergic to all three kinds of pollen. About 25 percent are allergic to both ragweed and grass pollen.

When seasonal rhinitis occurs in late spring or early summer it is sometimes called rose fever, another misnomer. Because roses are highly visible at just the time of year when grasses are pollinating, people naturally associate roses with summertime rhinitis. Actually, the pollen of colorful flowers—the much-maligned goldenrod as well as the rose—tends to be heavy and sticky, and is not easily transported by air. These plants are pollinated by insects, with the pollen designed to go from the flower to the insect. It is the virtually invisible pollen spread by the wind that most easily enters the nose and mouth, causing annoying respiratory symptoms.

On dry, windy days, pollen may fill the air and travel great distances. (Ragweed pollen can travel up to 500 miles!) Keep your home and car windows closed on such days, and use an air conditioner if possible.

If your hay fever is worse on rainy or damp days than on dry, sunny days, then you are more likely allergic to mold spores than to plant pollen. In general, seasonal mold allergies in the United States tend to be more common in the grain-growing states of the Midwest, for molds thrive on these plants. But allergenic molds are common in humid areas wherever there are trees and lawns, for mold grows well on dead leaves and grass cuttings. The allergic teenager who hates raking leaves or mowing lawns may not just be lazy—the jobs may leave him feeling sick. Another chore may be more appropriate for this youngster.

In the United States the most important molds are *Alternaria, Cladosporium* (also called *Hormodendrum*), and *Aspergillus*. Their spores, which appear in early spring, reach their highest levels on warm, humid summer days. The spores almost disappear with the first frost, but unless there is snow on the ground, there may still be mold spores in the air.

The Natural History of Allergic Rhinitis

Most people who develop allergic rhinitis do so before age 20, often between ages 12 and 15. The course of the disease for any given patient cannot be predicted because of the many variables involved, including pollen levels where the patient lives and works, emotional well-being of the patient, and so one. Typically, however, the disease persists for many years, with perennial rhinitis showing more staying power than the seasonal kinds. With seasonal rhinitis, one study has shown that, in a four-year period, about 1 in 20 women and 1 in 10 men recover and have no further symptoms.

Allergic rhinitis is often associated with asthma, and in some cases the asthma appears first. Rhinitis and asthma are in the triad of allergic atopic diseases, the third being eczema, or atopic dermatitis. Although patients often have two of the diseases, it is unusual to have all three.

Rhinitis Signs and Symptoms

As you can tell from its name, rhinitis (which means "inflammation of the nose") typically affects the nose. But in some patients, eye symptoms may dominate or the inflammation may move into the sinuses or ears.

In allergic rhinitis, nasal itching and serial sneezes (five or more sneezes in a row) are common. A watery secretion from the nose, with postnasal drip, is characteristic. An obstructed, "stuffy" nose is commonly reported. The nasal discharge can become quite copious, irritating the skin of the outer nose and upper lip. The patient tends to rub the nose and upper lip with a swiping gesture known as the "allergic salute."

Nasal obstruction, if it is more or less constant, can interfere with drainage of the paranasal sinuses, causing headache. The ache results from air pressure outside the sinuses as the absorption of air within the sinuses creates a negative pressure, or vacuum.

If nasal congestion blocks the Eustachian tube, you may get earaches, and your hearing will be muffled. Nasal congestion leads to loss of the senses of smell and taste.

Some patients report only itching and burning of the eyes, and sometimes a marked sensitivity to light. The sclera and conjunctiva, which form the lining of the eye, can become red and swollen (see chapter 11).

In chronic cases of rhinitis, especially in young children, the area around the eyes may be puffy and dark, as if the patient has two black eyes. These are called allergic shiners.

Itching of the throat, palate, and ears may provoke a patient to try to scratch the palate or throat with the tongue, which produces a clicking sound. One distinguished medical professor, ordinarily a very polite person, used to surprise students by putting his fingers in his mouth to scratch his throat—although only at the height of the allergy season.

The allergy may affect your mood, causing you to feel weak, sick, depressed, irritable, and tired. You may lose your appetite. Since these symptoms closely resemble those of clinical depression, the patient may end up in a psychotherapist's office or be treated with antidepressant medication. The diagnosis is especially difficult in the rare cases in which depression is virtually the only symptom. To discover the real culprit, the physician must look for a seasonal pattern or other environmental factor.

Some people with seasonal rhinitis suffer only at mid–pollen season. Others are so sensitive that they are reliable harbingers of spring. No sooner are the first grains of pollen in the air than they are on the phone to their allergists.

Some patients recover quickly as soon as the pollen season passes, but others suffer for several weeks longer. The nasal mucosa is primed, so that it will react to many different nonspecific stimuli, such as smoke or odors.

Perennial Allergic Rhinitis

The symptoms of perennial rhinitis tend to be less dramatic than those of seasonal rhinitis, except that obstruction by congestion is a far more prominent feature. Symptoms associated with such obstruction—including sinus headaches, chronic ear problems (especially in children), chronic sore throat caused by mouth breathing and postnasal drip, and itchiness of the nose and throat—are an important part of the picture.

Most often the person suffering from perennial rhinitis is allergic to one or more common substances in the environment—dust, indoor molds, or animal dander—the substances that in chapter 4 we advise you to clean out of your home. Occasionally a food is the cause. And in places like Southern California, where the pollen season lasts most of the year, so does the rhinitis.

The patient with perennial rhinitis develops very sensitive nasal mucosa, which may react to all sorts of nonspecific irritants, even changes in temperature. When pollen season comes around, the additional assault on the nasal tissues can make the symptoms much worse.

Diagnosis

In taking your history, in examining you, and in deciding what tests to run, the doctor will try to determine whether allergy is the main problem and what it is that you are allergic to. He or she will want to know if you have a family history of hay fever, eczema, or asthma. Expect a lot of questions relating to exactly when your symptoms appear and when they are at their worst, so if possible bring some notes on this subject (see chapter 3).

The doctor must be sure that no nonallergic condition, such as nasal polyps or a sinus infection unrelated to allergy, is responsible for your symptoms. He or she will try to find out if there is an asthmatic component to your illness and will ask about medicines you may be taking that may cause or worsen your symptoms.

Recurrent infections (colds) resemble allergic rhinitis, but usually the pattern of occurrence is different in that allergies tend to arise or get worse in the spring or summer and to last longer than colds. Also, with colds there is less itching and less repetitive sneezing; there is often fever; and the inside of the nose looks different than it does in patients with allergies.

Occasionally, especially with children, the physician will find something stuck up the nose, and removal of the foreign object provides a prompt happy ending.

Hypothyroidism (low levels of thyroid hormone) can produce nasal stuffiness. Hypothyroidism can be detected by a blood test. It is typically associated with fatigue and sometimes with hair loss.

Pregnancy is often accompanied by nasal stuffiness. This is normal.

Overuse of topical nasal decongestants causes chronic nasal congestion (rhinitis medicamentosa). A number of other drugs—including reserpine, alpha methyldopa, and beta blockers—can cause nasal congestion. Cocaine and some other illegal drugs cause a nasal condition similar to rhinitis medicamentosa.

Vasomotor rhinitis is very similar to perennial allergic rhinitis, but the cause is unknown. Symptoms are typically made worse by eating spicy food, by strong odors, or by sudden changes in temperature. Allergy tests (skin tests and RAST) will be negative (see chapter 3).

Another condition that tests negative for specific allergens is NARES (nonallergic rhinitis with eosinophilia). The patient seems to have allergic rhinitis, and a nasal smear test reveals an elevated count of eosinophils, blood cells that are associated with allergy. Many allergists feel that NARES is an allergic reaction to an unknown allergen or allergens in the environment.

Treatment

The management of allergic rhinitis consists of avoidance, medication, and immunotherapy (allergy shots).

Chapter 4 describes in detail what measures to take if your rhinitis is caused by allergens in your home. But in treating seasonal rhinitis, you must focus more on allergens from the great outdoors. If you can keep pollen and mold spores out of your home and office, the chances are that your hay fever will not be too severe. (If you do not improve much even when avoiding pollen and outdoor mold spores, one possibility that an allergist would investigate is whether you also have an asymptomatic sensitivity to one of the indoor allergens that is exacerbating your seasonal allergy.)

Usually the first step in controlling seasonal symptoms is to invest in an air conditioner, at least for the bedroom. If you have been working out of doors, gardening, raking leaves, or the like, wash your hair and put your clothing in the laundry before going to bed. You do not want to carry pollen and mold spores into your bedroom or bed.

Check out the plant life around your home. For years people with respiratory illnesses were sent to Tucson for their health. Soon, however, the fashion for growing Eastern lawns and gardens, in combination with the population's genetic inclination toward allergic sensitivities, produced a sort of chronic allergy emergency in that city, with half the population suffering from hay fever and/or asthma. Now laws prohibit the sale of mulberry and olive trees, and a fine of $300 per day may be assessed against the homeowner who lets a Bermuda grass lawn grow tall enough to flower.

In addition to olive and mulberry trees, acacia, juniper, elm, box elder, walnut, sycamore, ash, oak, birch, and maple are also heavy pollinators. However, the tree-pollination season comes early in spring and usually is relatively brief.

Late spring to early summer is the time when grasses begin to pollinate, with the duration of the season depending on location. In late summer and fall, plants of the ragweed family pollinate. These are the most problematic plants for allergy sufferers.

If you live in the country or near a vacant lot, and suffer from hay fever, be sure that you do not have a ragweed crop right on your doorstep. In the United States, the only almost-ragweed-free areas are the Pacific Coast, the southern tip of Florida, and northwest Maine.

Incidentally, alcoholic beverages sometimes cause increased allergic sensitivity, so when the pollen count is high, you may want to keep your alcohol consumption low.

Moving to a different part of the country in order to avoid exposure to the plants and molds to which you are sensitive is rarely worthwhile and often an expensive disappointment. You may well develop new allergies to the plants—even desert plants—in your new home region. However, if you have successfully visited in a region for several months and you always feel better there, this may be the exception to the rule.

As for medication or immunization, your doctor should be willing to take the time to explain the costs and benefits of a variety of approaches to reducing rhinitis symptoms. Unless the rhinitis is associated with some other, more serious, condition, such as asthma or perhaps sinus disease, you can safely begin with a minimalist approach to treatment, working up to more expensive treatment or immunization only if necessary.

Relatively new and very helpful medications include the non-soporific antihistamines (which may be combined with a decongestant) and cromolyn and topical corticosteroid nasal sprays (see chapter 5). Remember, it is extremely important to use the sprays only as directed. Also, the antihistamines, as well as cromolyn and corticosteroid sprays, work best when started in advance of an outbreak of allergy symptoms; they (especially the sprays) are essentially preventives.

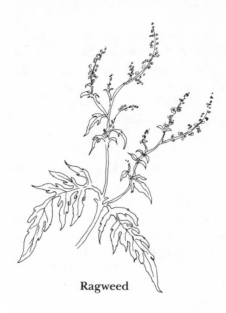

Ragweed

Immediate relief from nasal stuffiness can be obtained by use of normal saline solution (⅛ teaspoon of salt in 8 ounces of water). With a bulb syringe, irrigate the nasal passages to wash away mucus and allergens. Do one nostril at a time, and allow the water to flow in gently. Don't force the water through the congested areas. Saline solution can also be used to wash out itchy, inflamed eyes.

Most often, if you take steps to reduce exposure to the allergens that provoke your rhinitis, a moderate amount of medication can bring adequate relief. But if you have a number of allergies and year-round symptoms, then you might reasonably consider immunotherapy for a more thoroughgoing improvement. The decision whether or not to take this step may turn on exactly which allergens affect you (as revealed by skin and/or blood tests). Immunization is achieved more readily for some allergens than others, and your doctor should discuss this with you.

Also, for various reasons, some patients cannot tolerate the drugs normally used to treat rhinitis, and so immunotherapy and very strict avoidance of allergens must be attempted.

Pollination Seasons

The following summary of pollination seasons lists general pollination dates for significant varieties of plants in the United States. The seasonal dates will vary from region to region and will also change from year to year, depending on weather conditions. Finally, you may be allergic to plants in your region that are not listed here. So if you have hay fever, take the time to do a little botanical investigation of your neighborhood. Your local health officer, botanical gardens, or forestry service should be able to help you to identify troublesome plants.

In many places, the pollination period for trees overlaps with that of grass and that of grass overlaps with that of ragweed. Therefore, the many people who are allergic to more than one type of plant are susceptible to a double whammy in summer and early fall. Molds (not listed here) also are prevalent in summer and fall, especially in damp weather.

If you are allergic to one grass, you are probably allergic to several. Related antigenically are timothy, orchard grass, redtop, sweet vernal grass, rye, fescue, and Johnsongrass. Bermuda grass belongs to a different family. It is usually found in Southern states, and if kept trimmed, as in a lawn, it will not pollinate. But it also grows wild along roadways and in fields, where, of course, it does pollinate.

The pollination seasons listed below are generally for the southern part of each region; they will occur later in the more northerly sections.

North Atlantic States

Connecticut, Maine, Massachusetts, New Jersey, New Hampshire, New York, Pennsylvania, Rhode Island, and Vermont:

Trees. Trees in this region pollinate from March through June, with box elder and maple pollinating early (March through May) and oak being the latest (May and June). Other significant trees are ash, birch, cottonwood, elm, hickory, poplar, sycamore, and walnut.

Grasses. Grasses (many of which are grown as hay) pollinate from May through July. They include bromegrass, fescue,

Johnsongrass, Junegrass (Kentucky bluegrass), orchard grass, redtop, rye, timothy, velvet grass, and vernal grass.

Weeds. Early-pollinating weeds are plantain (not the banana plant but an herb of the genus *Plantago*) and dock (sorrel) (May through July). Late pollinators are cocklebur, lamb's-quarters, pigweed, and ragweed (August through October).

Mid-Atlantic States

Delaware, District of Columbia, Maryland, North Carolina, and Virginia:

Trees. Trees pollinate from February through May, with box elder, maple, and elm being the earliest and hickory and pecan the latest. Others include ash, birch, cedar, cottonwood, juniper, oak, poplar, sycamore, and walnut.

Grasses. May through July is the grass-pollinating season. The following grasses are important: Bermuda grass, Johnsongrass, Junegrass (Kentucky bluegrass), orchard grass, redtop, rye, timothy, and vernal grass.

Weeds. Among weeds, dock (sorrel) is an early pollinator (May through July), along with plantain (May through August). Cocklebur, lamb's-quarters, pigweed, and ragweed pollinate from August through October.

South Atlantic States

Florida, Georgia, and South Carolina; the southern tip of Florida is one of the few places in the United States that does not have much ragweed. Plants characteristic of subtropical Florida to which people are allergic include palm trees, Brazilian pepper trees, bayberry, and melaleuca trees, which pollinate from December through April. Grasses pollinate year-round in subtropical Florida.

Trees. In this region generally, trees pollinate from January through May, with cedar and juniper being early pollinators and walnut pollinating in May. Privet pollinates all year. Other trees of interest to the allergy-prone include ash, birch, box elder, cottonwood, elm, hickory, maple, oak, pecan, pine, poplar, and sycamore.

Grasses. Grasses pollinate from March through October. They include Bermuda grass, canary grass, fescue, Johnsongrass, Junegrass (Kentucky bluegrass), redtop, rye, timothy, and vernal grass. The subtropical grasses include Bahia grass and salt grass. As mentioned, at the tip of Florida grasses pollinate year-round.

Weeds. Weed pollination starts in May and continues through October. The significant weeds include dock (sorrel) and plantain (early pollinators), as well as cocklebur, lamb's-quarters, pigweed, ragweed, and sagebrush, which pollinate from July through October.

Greater Ohio Valley

Indiana, Kentucky, Ohio, Tennessee, and West Virginia:

Trees. In this region, the earliest-pollinating tree is elm (February through April). Hickory trees pollinate as late as June. Others, which pollinate in the spring, include ash, birch, box elder, cottonwood, elm, maple, oak, poplar, sycamore, and walnut.

Grasses. Pollination of grasses is from April through July, with grass plants including Bermuda grass, fescue, Johnsongrass, Junegrass (Kentucky bluegrass), redtop, rye, and timothy.

Weeds. The peak weed-pollination season is August through October, with plantain pollinating as early as May and the all-important ragweed pollinating from August through October. Others include amaranth, cocklebur, dock (sorrel), kochia, lamb's-quarters, pigweed, Russian thistle, sagebrush, and water hemp.

South Central States

Alabama, Arkansas, Louisiana, and Mississippi:

Trees. Tree pollination starts in February and runs through May. The significant trees include ash, box elder, cedar, cottonwood, elm, hackberry, hickory, juniper, maple, oak, pecan, poplar, and sycamore.

Grasses. April through September is grass-pollination season, with the following important plants represented: Bermuda grass, Johnsongrass, Junegrass (Kentucky bluegrass), orchard grass, redtop, rye, and timothy.

Weeds. In May through July, plantain and dock (sorrel) pollinate, followed by kochia and Russian thistle in June through August. In August through October the pollinators include careless weed, cocklebur, lamb's-quarters, marsh elder, pigweed, poverty weed, ragweed, and sagebrush.

Midwestern States

Illinois, Iowa, Michigan, Minnesota, Missouri, and Wisconsin:

Trees. The elm opens the season, beginning pollination in February. The main months of tree pollination are March through June, with the following represented: alder, ash, box elder, birch, cedar, cottonwood, hickory, maple, oak, poplar, sycamore, and walnut.

Grasses. Grass-pollination season is April through August. Keep in mind that dates are given for the southern part of the region; the pollination season runs about a month later in the north. The main grasses to which people are likely to be sensitive are Bermuda grass, bromegrass, Canada bluegrass, canary grass, corn, fescue, Johnsongrass, Junegrass (Kentucky bluegrass), orchard grass, redtop, rye, and timothy.

Weeds. In May through July, plantain and dock (sorrel) pollinate, followed by kochia and Russian thistle in June through August. In August through October the pollinators include amaranth, chenopod, careless weed, cocklebur, lamb's-quarters, marsh elder, Mexican firebush, pigweed, poverty weed, and ragweed.

The Great Plains

Kansas, Nebraska, North Dakota, and South Dakota:

Trees. Pollination begins in March and goes into June, with the main trees being alder, ash, birch, box elder, cedar, cottonwood, elm, hickory, maple, oak, poplar, pussy willow, and walnut.

Grasses. Grass-pollination season is May through July. The most important grasses are bromegrass, fescue, Junegrass (Kentucky bluegrass), quack grass, redtop, rye, timothy, Western and crested wheatgrass.

Weeds. Plantain and dock (sorrel) pollinate in May through July. Ragweed and other important weeds pollinate July through October. They include amaranth, cocklebur, lamb's-quarters, marsh elder, Mexican firebush, pigweed, poverty weed, Russian thistle, sagebrush, and water hemp.

Southwestern Grasslands

Oklahoma and Texas:

Trees. Tree-pollination season lasts from February through April. Important trees include ash, box elder, cedar, cottonwood, elm, hickory, juniper, mesquite, mulberry, oak, pecan, poplar, walnut, and willow.

Grasses. Grass-pollination season is April through August. The most important grasses are Bermuda grass, fescue, Johnsongrass, Junegrass (Kentucky bluegrass), orchard grass, quack grass, redtop, rye, and timothy.

Weeds. Pollination season is May through October. Ragweed pollinates August through October. Other weeds include careless weed, cocklebur, dock (sorrel), kochia, lamb's-quarters, marsh elder, pigweed, plantain, Russian thistle, and sagebrush.

Rocky Mountain States

Arizona (mountainous), Colorado, Idaho (mountainous), Montana, New Mexico, Utah, and Wyoming:

Trees. The pollination season begins as early as December in the southern part of this region (for the mountain cedar). It lasts through June. In addition to the mountain cedar, other significant trees are alder, ash, aspen, birch, box elder, cedar, cottonwood, elm, hickory, juniper, mesquite, mulberry, oak, olive, pine, poplar, and willow.

Grasses. Pollination of grasses is April through September (April through August in the south and May through September in the north). The following grasses are represented: Bermuda grass, bromegrass, fescue, Junegrass (Kentucky bluegrass), orchard grass, quack grass, redtop, rye, and timothy.

Weeds. Pollination season is May through October. Ragweed pollinates July through September. Other weeds include amaranth, careless weed, cocklebur, lamb's-quarters, marsh elder, pigweed, plantain, Russian thistle, sagebush, saltbush, and sugar beet.

Southwestern Desert

Arizona (desert) and Southern California:

Trees. The pollination season begins in January and lasts through May. Important trees include ash, cedar, cottonwood, cypress, elm, juniper, mesquite, oak, poplar, and sycamore.

Grasses. Pollination of grasses is virtually year-round. The following grasses are represented: Bermuda grass, bromegrass, canary grass, Junegrass (Kentucky bluegrass), and rye.

Weeds. Pollination season is May into November. Ragweed pollinates in March and April and in September and October. Other weeds include careless weed, lamb's-quarters, pigweed, Russian thistle, sagebrush, and saltbush.

Intermountain Western States

Idaho (southern) and Nevada:

Trees. The pollination season is February through May. Significant trees are alder, ash, birch, box elder, cedar, cottonwood, elm, juniper, mesquite, poplar, and willow.

Grasses. Pollination of grasses is May through July. The following grasses are represented: Bermuda grass, bromegrass, fescue, Junegrass (Kentucky bluegrass), orchard grass, quack grass, redtop, rye, salt grass, and timothy.

Weeds. Pollination season is primarily July through October, with dock (sorrel) and saltbush beginning pollination early (in May). Other weeds include cocklebur, kochia, lamb's-quarters, Mexican firebush, ragweed, Russian thistle, and sagebrush.

California (Nondesert) and the Pacific Northwest

California, Oregon, and Washington:

Trees. Pollination begins in February and lasts through June. Major trees are acacia, alder, ash, birch, box elder, cottonwood, elm, hazelnut, poplar, sycamore, walnut, and willow.

Grasses. Pollination of grasses occurs from February through November (primarily May through August in the north). The following grasses are represented: Bermuda grass, bromegrass, canary grass, fescue, Johnsongrass, Junegrass (Kentucky bluegrass), oats, orchard grass, redtop, rye, and timothy.

Weeds. Pollination season is May through October. There is very little ragweed here, although it does exist. Other weeds include careless weed, cocklebur, dock (sorrel), kochia, lamb's-quarters, pigweed, plantain, Russian thistle, sagebrush, saltbush, and sheep sorrel.

Alaska

Airborne allergens are not a great problem here. There is a tree-pollination season from March through June, overlapping with a brief time of grass pollination in certain areas in June and July.

The most important trees are alder, birch, and willow. Others include aspen, cedar, hemlock, pine, poplar, and spruce. The grasses include Junegrass (Kentucky bluegrass), orchard grass, redtop, and timothy.

Hawaii

Pollen season is essentially all year.

Trees. A few trees contribute sufficient airborne pollen to be a problem. These include acacia and eucalyptus.

Grasses. Significant grasses relative to allergy include Bermuda grass, corn, finger grass, Johnsongrass, Junegrass (Kentucky bluegrass), love grass, redtop, and sorghum.

Weeds. Pollen of English plantain, lamb's-quarters, and pigweed is a problem in some places.

11

Sinuses, Ears, and Eyes

Allergies, especially allergic rhinitis, can be associated with chronic or acute infection or inflammation of the sinuses, ears, or eyes. When a patient has chronic sinus disease or earaches, often it is not initially clear whether allergies play a role or not.

Both allergists and ear, nose, and throat specialists treat disorders of the sinuses and ears, and sometimes eyes, as do doctors with a wider practice, such as pediatricians and internists. (The technical term for an ear, nose, and throat doctor is otolaryngologist. ENT is the popular shorthand designation.)

Ideally, there should be cooperation among different specialists. For example, if sinusitis keeps recurring after antibiotic treatment, tests for allergic sensitivities should be done to see whether allergic reactions may be causing blockage of the sinuses, thereby contributing to the development of infection. Similarly, an allergist who is treating sinus disease without much luck should consider referring the patient to a sinus specialist. In some cases, for instance, surgery is needed to help the sinuses to drain.

As a patient or as a parent of a patient, be aware that it is appropriate to seek a second opinion if a health problem continues. Often it is helpful to go to a doctor in a different specialty.

Nasal Polyps

One condition for which it is important to see both an allergist and an ENT is the presence of nasal polyps. The symptoms, usually severe enough that the person realizes a visit to the doctor is needed, are typically chronic nasal congestion, headaches, sinus aches, loss of the senses of smell and taste, and recurrent ear congestion or infection.

Luckily polyps are relatively uncommon, because they are troubling and sometimes serious. They are usually associated with nasal disease or asthma, often asthma combined with aspirin sensitivity. If you have asthma and polyps, it is very likely that you are also allergic to aspirin and to other nonsteroidal anti-inflammatory drugs as well. Asthma attacks caused by aspirin allergy are often exceptionally severe when nasal polyps are present.

Polyps afflict people with the atopic allergic diseases (allergic rhinitis, asthma, and eczema) more than they do the general population and are twice as common in men as in women. The great majority of polyps occur after age 40. In a child under age ten, the growth of polyps is highly suggestive of cystic fibrosis.

Polyps are growths, typically benign, off the side walls of the nasal passages or in the sinus cavities. Malignancy is relatively rare, although it is much more likely if the polyps appear only on one side of the nose or if they bleed easily. But in all cases, the possibility of a malignancy should be ruled out by an ENT; this is mandatory if the polyps are on one side only.

It is not clear exactly what causes polyps to grow, except that they seem to do so when patients are allergic or when there is some recurrent infection or irritation of the nose and sinuses.

Formerly, surgical removal was the standard treatment, but since polyps tend to grow back, even after surgery, it is usually better to try less intrusive medical treatment first. Today we have effective treatment that is not so aggressive. The most useful medical treatment is with topical nasal steroids. Antihistamines and decongestants do not help. Also, since polyps are so often linked with allergies, it is a good idea to see an allergist to determine whether or not you have allergic sensitivities. Sometimes, good environmental control of the allergens in your home is treatment enough to control the allergic factor in the condition. In other cases, immunotherapy (allergy shots) may be helpful. The latter two interventions will not reverse the polyps but can decrease the chances they will regrow following steroid treatment or surgery.

If steroid treatment does not work, surgery may be needed, but immediately after surgery it is important to proceed with medical treatment to prevent the polyps from growing back. Allergy treatment should also begin if allergies have been detected.

Sinusitis

Sinus disease is a much more common condition than most people realize. It is more common, for example, than arthritis.

Sometimes people fail to recognize sinus pain as an indication of a sinus infection for the simple reason that they are not sure where their sinuses are.

The sinuses are spaces in the skull bone surrounding the inner nose; each sinus has an opening that drains into the nose. These openings are called the ostia.

There are four pairs of sinuses. The frontal sinuses are above the eyebrows; the maxillary sinuses are in the cheekbones below the eyes; the ethmoidal sinuses are beneath the sides of the nose; and the sphenoidal sinuses lie deeper in the head, behind the ethmoidal sinuses.

Only the maxillary and sphenoidal sinuses are present at birth. The frontal sinuses develop at about age five, and in some individuals they do not develop at all. The sphenoids appear at about age nine.

The precise evolutionary function of the sinuses is not known. Perhaps their main purpose is to lighten the head so that it is easier to walk upright. (Apes, who have heavier skulls than humans, do not have sinuses.) Possibly sinuses play a role in smelling, in the production of mucus, and in phonation (forming sounds).

Sinus Disease

The cause of sinus disease is mucus congestion in the sinus cavities, setting the stage for infection. The sinuses are lined with a mucus-producing membrane and cilia, or tiny waving hairs,

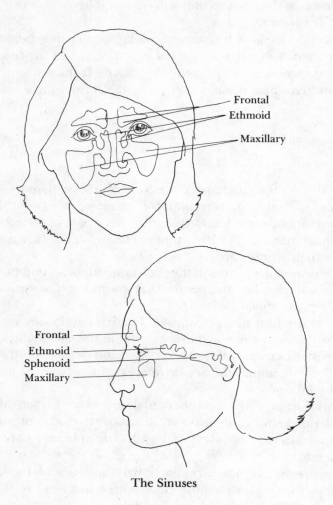

Frontal
Ethmoid

Maxillary

Frontal
Ethmoid
Sphenoid
Maxillary

The Sinuses

which move a thin layer of mucus over the lining of the sinuses. Bacteria and particles of dust, pollen, and so on are normally trapped in the mucus and propelled out of the sinuses into the nasal cavity.

Interference with this normal flow of mucus can cause sinusitis. The interference can be blockage of the ostia, so that the sinuses cannot drain; or limitation on the movement of the cilia; or an overproduction of mucus.

Blockage of the ostia is the most common cause of sinusitis. It occurs most commonly after an upper respiratory infection (a cold) or from an allergic reaction causing inflammation and swelling of the nasal tissues. Other causes of blockage are over-use of topical nasal decongestants, swollen adenoids, a deviated septum (a shifting of the cartilage that runs down the center of the nose), polyps, and tumors or foreign bodies. Smoking cigarettes interferes with action of the cilia and predisposes the smoker to sinus infection, and some types of immune-system deficiency may predispose a person to develop sinusitis.

Chronic and Acute Sinusitis

Sinusitis appears in two forms: chronic and acute. Typically, acute sinusitis arises after an upper-respiratory-tract infection, although only about 1 in 200 upper-respiratory-tract infections leads to acute sinusitis.

Acute sinusitis usually sets in after you have had a cold for several days and your nasal discharge becomes yellow or dark green, thick, and perhaps foul-smelling. You feel persistent pain high in your cheeks, around and behind the eyes, and in the forehead over your eyes. If you lean forward, the pain is often worse. You may find spots that are tender to the touch. Sometimes the sinuses even puff out slightly. You may also have a fever.

If these symptoms appear, you should see a doctor promptly. Occasionally, although very rarely, sinusitis can spread to the area around the eyes (in an orbital abscess) or into the bone around the sinuses (osteomyelitis). Even more rarely, the infection may spread to the brain (as a brain abscess).

Visible, palpable swelling of the sinuses occurs more often in children than adults. The swelling will be around or near the eyes. But usually the presentation of acute sinusitis is less dramatic in children than in adults. The youngster may have a purulent nasal discharge and bad breath, but the most important symptom may be a cough. A nasty, persistent cough, whether or not the other symptoms are present, may mean that a child has sinus disease. One seven-year-old boy recently treated turned out to have this problem. He had a nagging, dry cough, but a chest X ray showed nothing. The parents were wondering whether to try a psychiatrist or an allergist. They decided on an allergist. Sinus X rays showed a bad infection.

In chronic sinusitis, the symptoms are generally undramatic. The pain is dull rather than sharp, and there is a feeling of fullness from congestion in the sinuses. Often the patient has a steady postnasal drip, which can cause coughing and an irritated, sore throat. The breath may be fetid. This unpleasant but generally not life-threatening disease affects some 31 million people in the United States, according to the Department of Health and Human Services.

Nevertheless, chronic sinusitis can occasionally become a serious health problem, especially for asthmatics. Sinus inflammation and congestion can make asthma much worse. Any asthmatic who is not doing well should have sinus X rays or even CAT scans done at some point to determine if sinus disease is involved.

Treatment

The treatment of an acute sinus infection includes pain medication, topical or oral decongestants to help unblock the ostia and promote drainage, hot compresses for the front of the face over the sinuses to stimulate blood flow and drainage, increased fluid intake, and, most important, antibiotics.

The antibiotic usually used is amoxicillin. If you are allergic to penicillin drugs, there are a number of other drugs that may work, including erythromycin, doxycycline, or trimethoprim with sulfamethoxazole.

The treatment must continue longer than for many other sorts of infections. A course of three weeks or more may be needed to ensure eradication of the infection. Follow-up sinus X rays may be needed to be certain that the infection is gone.

Chronic infections typically respond less well to antibiotics. Often lavage (washing out) of the sinuses by an ENT is necessary. Then antibiotics may be used more effectively. Sometimes intranasal steroids are helpful in reducing swelling that is blocking the ostia and in promoting sinus drainage.

If you have chronic sinusitis, you should see an allergist to determine if you have allergies that are causing rhinitis, which in turn is causing the sinus disease. Frequently, allergies do underlie sinus disease.

If you have been suffering from a sinus infection relating to allergies, medication is also likely to be needed, including antihistamines, decongestants, nasal steroids, or cromolyn. If your allergies cause severe or year-round symptoms, immunotherapy (allergy shots) may be required.

Although you can sometimes successfully self-medicate mild allergies, if you have sinus disease you should see a doctor. The infection should be eradicated. If antihistamines are needed, you will probably want a prescription for one of the newer, non-sedating antihistamines.

Sometimes surgery is needed for stubborn sinus infections in which the infected sinuses simply do not drain adequately despite vigorous medical treatment. There are many surgical techniques, but the ordinary goal is to provide an opening (a "window") from the sinuses into the nasal cavity.

Surgery should be followed up by aggressive medical treatment to prevent recurrence of the infection. If you are allergic, probably both immunotherapy and strict environmental control of your exposure to allergens will be needed.

Ear Infections

Earaches and ear blockage may be caused by numerous conditions, including allergic rhinitis. Serous otitis media (a persistent or recurring collection of fluid in the middle ear) is especially common in childhood, affecting 50 percent of all children at some point in their young lives.

With the advent of antibiotics, serous otitis and middle-ear infections have not generally been regarded with much concern. But recent evidence suggests that ear ailments in infants and toddlers may cause a loss of hearing at critical stages of language development.

These early-childhood ear disorders can be related to allergy. Sometimes, though rarely, a milk allergy contributes to the problem. Whatever the cause, every parent should discuss with a pediatrician what signs indicate a possible hearing blockage. If language development or responsiveness is impaired, the reason may be a hearing problem related to chronic serous otitis media or recurring ear infections.

The reason that children, particularly under age seven, are more prone to ear blockage and infections than adults is that the smaller size of the child's skull sets the Eustachian tube at a different angle than in adults. The Eustachian tube runs from

Allergies

the middle ear to the nasal cavity, and in children it is not set as vertically as in adults. It is more prone to obstruction, and fluid from the nose also may leak into the ear more readily, especially when the child is lying on his or her back.

In adulthood, the likelihood that the ears will collect fluid or become infected varies from individual to individual, but it is generally less than in childhood. Chronic ear infections, especially on one side only, should be evaluated by an ENT specialist. The cause may be a malignant tumor. These tumors tend to be more common among Asians. Serous otitis is quite common among Eskimos and American Indians.

The simple collection of fluid in the ears, without infection, is experienced mainly as a sense of fullness in the ears, sometimes with popping and a loss of hearing. (The Eustachian tube serves to equalize air pressure between the middle ear and the outside air. When the change in pressure is sudden, as when ascending in an elevator, popping occurs. Chewing gum helps to open the tube, which is why gum used to be handed out in airplanes during takeoffs and landings, when rapid pressure changes may happen.)

If the collected fluid helps an infection become established, pain and usually fever result and antibiotic treatment is needed. Sometimes even surgery is required. Adenoids may be obstructing the tubes, and they may have to be removed. Sometimes it is necessary to create a drainage passage surgically.

Chronic allergic rhinitis may contribute to chronic serous otitis in children and adults. Although allergic rhinitis varies in seriousness and does not always require aggressive treatment, it should be taken seriously if it is associated with ear problems.

Finally, there have been some reports of foods producing symptoms resembling Ménière's disease. This disease involves poor function of the balance mechanism of the inner ear; the patient experiences vertigo (a sensation that the room is spinning), hearing loss, painful ringing in the ears, and sometimes nausea and vomiting. This disease, which affects some 7 million Americans, was identified in 1861 by Prosper Ménière in Paris, France. Recently, it has been theorized in the *Journal of the American Medical Association* that this disorder afflicted Vincent van Gogh. But there is no clear evidence that food allergy plays a role in Ménière's disease. The connection is still only speculative.

Eyes

Allergies often lead to symptoms involving the eye. Indeed, allergic rhinitis is sometimes apparent almost solely in eye symptoms, such as itching and swelling. But luckily, allergy-based eye problems are rarely so serious as to threaten eyesight.

Allergy symptoms may arise very noticeably in the eyes because the conjuctiva contains mast cells. The conjunctiva is the mucous membrane covering the front of the eye and the inner part of the eyelids. Mast cells carry histamine and other chemical mediators that cause the typical allergy reactions of swelling, inflammation, and itching.

When an allergen, such as a particle of pollen or dander, links up with an allergy antibody and a mast cell, then histamine and the other mediators are rapidly released. For example, if a pollen-allergic person is exposed to, say, a heavy dose of ragweed pollen, the eyes may begin to itch, burn, water, and sting. They also may become very light-sensitive, and swelling may occur.

Treatment is essentially the same as for allergic rhinitis. Antihistamines may be sufficient, or the full spectrum of medication and desensitization may be needed.

Recently, optic cromolyn has become available. It prevents the release of allergy mediators from the mast cells, but it ordinarily takes several days to a week of regular use to begin to work. It is best to begin using optic cromolyn before exposure—for example, before the onset of the season in which allergy symptoms usually develop.

Severe cases may require the use of topical steroids, but this should be decided by an ophthalmologist (eye specialist), as steroid use may be associated with the development of glaucoma, cataracts, or infections.

Atopic dermatitis (eczema) also can involve the eyes, in which case the name of the disorder is atopic keratoconjunctivitis. Red lesions appear on the eyelids, followed by crusting and scaling. In severe cases, the eyes produce excess tears, and patients become so sensitive to light that they have difficulty opening their eyes in full daylight. Ultimately, the cornea may be damaged or cataracts may form.

The treatment is with steroids, under the direction of an ophthalmologist. Optic cromolyn may be of some help. If infections arise in the lesions, antibiotic treatment may be needed.

Obviously, if allergy is contributing to this condition, it should be dealt with promptly to avert the serious complications.

Children often develop a seasonal type of conjunctivitis, arising in spring and summer, with very intense itching of the eyes and sensitivity to light. In this disease, called vernal keratoconjunctivitis, there is a characteristic cobblestone appearance of the conjunctiva under the eyelids.

Sometimes the condition lasts year-round. Happily, it usually disappears at puberty, although adults, too, may be affected. Males are three times as likely as females to suffer from vernal keratoconjunctivitis.

The cause of the disease is not known for certain, but there are strong clues that it is related to allergy. First is the seasonal pattern. Second, eosinophils are present in the conjunctival fluid. (These are the blood cells whose number is characteristically elevated in allergy.) Also, most patients have other atopic illnesses, such as allergic rhinitis or asthma.

Again, the most effective treatment is with topical steroids. Even though the patients may be very young, they must be followed by an ophthalmologist and checked for glaucoma. Use of steroids like medrysone and fluorometholone, which are poorly absorbed, is advisable, since these are less likely to produce glaucoma.

Other drugs of variable benefit include vasoconstrictors, cromolyn, antihistamines, and acetylcysteine (a drug used to treat lung diseases).

Wearing contact lenses, especially soft lenses, is often associated with an itchy eye condition called giant papillary conjunctivitis. Often the patient must give up use of the lenses. Sometimes a change of lens type or more frequent cleaning of the lenses prevents the condition from recurring.

Women in particular are prone to contact dermatitis of the eyelids as a result of an allergic reaction to cosmetics or other substances. The eyelid blisters and then thickens and turns red. The eyes itch. The conjunctiva may also be affected, with tearing and redness of the eyes.

The cause of contact dermatitis on the eyelids may be a sensitivity to: (1) makeup or skin cleansers; (2) eye medications, including prescription drugs such as neomycin or antiviral agents; (3) solutions for wetting or cleaning contact lenses, especially if they contain thimerosal and some other anti-infective substances; and (4) airborne agents, including hair spray, substances found in the workplace, pollen, and nail polish (when the person touches the lids with the polished nails).

Diagnosis may require patch testing to determine what substance is causing the problem, but if you are a contact-lens wearer, the most obvious first step is to use a different lens solution or to switch to thermal rather than chemical disinfection of the lenses.

Local corticosteroid creams or drops will probably help, but again, *never use these steroid medications without the supervision of an eye doctor.*

12

Skin Disorders

Hives and Angioedema

Hives are an annoying nuisance, the acute variety affecting more than 20 percent of people at some point in their lives. The condition, technically called urticaria, is ordinarily harmless although uncomfortable. But you should always try to determine what has caused hives to appear, because sometimes they signal the development of a dangerous sensitivity to a food or drug that might lead in the future to an anaphylactic reaction. Sometimes they may be a sign of exposure to a toxic substance.

A hive is a relatively small, itchy, red, elevated spot that resembles a mosquito bite. The hive may be just one or two millimeters to several centimeters in diameter, and can appear anywhere on the body.

You may suffer from just one hive or many. Hives tend to come and go in a matter of one to several hours. If a single hive lasts for more than 24 hours, notify your doctor. Such persistent lesions may be a sign of vasculitis, which is a swelling of the blood vessels. There are several different types of vasculitis, but all require medical attention.

An attack of hives may last from several hours to several days or even weeks. Hives that persist for longer than six weeks are categorized as chronic.

Both chronic and acute urticaria may or may not be allergic in nature. Acute outbreaks of hives, however, are quite often traceable to specific allergies, such as an allergy to drugs or to foods. Chronic hives are less likely to be related to allergy.

Angioedema is similar to hives in that it involves swelling and may be caused by allergies. But in angioedema the swelling is subcutaneous—that is, it occurs deeper under the skin—and there is usually little or no itching.

Women develop angioedema more frequently than men do, and the condition often arises in adulthood. It may occur in conjunction with hives or alone. The swelling lasts for from a few hours to three days (in hereditary angioedema).

Angioedema without hives most often involves the face, tongue, extremities (hands and feet), or genitals. When hives are present, the angioedema may affect the tongue and pharynx. In anaphylactic reactions and in the hereditary form of angio-edema, the respiratory tract may be affected.

Any kind of choking reaction or swelling of the throat should be brought to a doctor's attention, even if the episode passes safely. The next time the reaction may be more severe. Your doctor may prescribe an EpiPen for you to carry; this is a device containing a dose of injectable epinephrine (Adrenalin).

The physiological mechanisms underlying allergic hives and angioedema are essentially the same as in all other allergic re-actions. But, as you might expect in reactions involving the skin, the most active mast cells (releasing histamine and other chem-ical allergy mediators) are located primarily in the skin or in tissue just under the skin.

The redness of the skin is caused by swelling of the blood vessels and by blood leaking from the smallest vessels (the cap-illaries). Both effects are due to the vasodilation caused by his-tamine and its chemical relatives.

In most cases, the release of histamine in outbreaks of hives and angioedema is not caused by the standard allergic linkage of allergen–to–IgE antibody–to–mast cell, although involve-ment of the immune system apart from IgE action has been demonstrated in some cases. In many instances the mechanisms producing hives and angioedema are not fully known.

About 80 percent of cases of chronic urticaria are classified as idiopathic urticaria; *idiopathic* means that the cause of the hives is not known.

The "physical allergies" include attacks of hives brought on by cold, pressure, sunlight, and other factors.

Frankly, there is still much to learn with respect to both the causes and mechanisms of urticaria. It is known, however, that alcohol, stress, and hormonal fluctuations during the menstrual cycle all can aggravate urticaria, no matter what the underlying cause. Other factors are outlined below.

Causes of Hives and Combined Hives and Angioedema

1. Drugs, foods, and food additives. In an acute outbreak of hives, a common culprit is a drug, especially penicillin, the related cephalosporin drugs, and other antibiotics. In very sensitive patients, even the minute amounts of antibiotics present in some meats and dairy products can cause hives. The reaction can appear within seconds of ingesting the drug or up to ten days later. The attack may last up to two months after the drug is stopped.

Ampicillin can cause very delayed hives, at times first appearing several weeks after the drug is taken and sometimes lasting a few months. Many other drugs are on the roster of usual suspects, including sulfonylurea drugs (used for treating diabetes), many diuretics, and certain local anesthetics.

Aspirin can cause hives or aggravate existing hives, but sensitivity to aspirin is not a true allergy; it is, instead, an intolerance that includes other anti-inflammatories, such as indomethacin and ibuprofen. If you get hives from anti-inflammatory drugs, you may also be sensitive to the food-coloring additive tartrazine (FD&C Yellow #5). Other additives that may provoke hives are salicylates and benzoic acid (see chapter 7).

This cross-sensitivity to aspirin and additives can be the cause of both acute hives and perhaps up to 10 percent of the cases of chronic hives. The usual method of pinpointing the offending substances is to restrict food intake for a week to a canned, prescription, additive-free nutritional supplement and see if the hives go away. Unfortunately, there is no skin or blood test for this sensitivity.

Because aspirin and other anti-inflammatories so often aggravate hives even if they are not the actual cause of the condition, it is probably just as well to avoid these drugs if you have chronic hives. If you need medication, consult with your physician. In the place of these drugs, you may find that you can use choline trisalicylate (Trilisate) and related drugs.

Food allergies also commonly cause acute outbreaks of hives and angioedema, but they can be blamed for chronic hives much less often.

When a food is the suspected cause, the suspicion can sometimes be confirmed by RAST and skin testing. With acute hives, food in the same family as the offending food may have to be eliminated. For instance, if you are allergic to one kind of bony fish, you may be allergic to all bony fish (see chapter 7).

With chronic urticaria, a single food is rarely the cause. Testing for allergy to a vast number of foods may merely yield false positives, which can be a considerable waste of time and money. Instead, you can try keeping a food diary listing all the foods you eat so that an allergenic food can be identified. In some cases, patients are asked to go on a restricted diet, starting with rice, lamb (or chicken), and water for three days. Gradually new foods will be introduced to see if they cause the hives (see chapter 7).

2. Exercise. Exercise-induced hives can be a danger sign, indicating the onset of anaphylaxis. The mast cells are involved, but the cause is not really understood. In some patients, the risk exists only if they have eaten within a few hours of exercising; with others, the risk is dependent upon their having eaten certain specific foods, such as shrimp or celery. For these latter patients, neither eating the food alone nor exercising alone is risky, but doing both can be dangerous.

In some people, the heating of the body during exercise produces very small itchy hives, sometimes associated with wheezing but not anaphylaxis. See the section on cholinergic urticaria below.

3. Underlying illness. Hives sometimes signal an underlying infection. The possible underlying conditions range from mild viral infections to cancer.

In rare cases, hepatitis B may present as hives. This is a relatively recent discovery, and in the past the association of urticaria and hepatitis was something of a surprise when it occurred. Today, if a patient develops hives and undefined illness, the diagnosis of hepatitis should come to mind more readily.

As mentioned above, vasculitis (inflammation of the blood vessels) may be a cause of hives, especially when individual hives tend to persist in one location. A variety of other underlying bacterial, viral, and fungal infections may cause hives, as may infestation with parasitic worms.

An adverse reaction to a blood transfusion may involve hives. Serum sickness from drugs also may result in hives.

There are also disorders of the mast cells that lead to hives.

4. Physical allergies. These are allergic-type reactions to a physical stimulus such as heat or cold that produce hives.

Cold sensitivity. Some people suffer hives and angioedema when their skin is exposed to cold. Often the symptoms get worse when the area is warmed again. Frequently, the reaction is limited to contact with cold air, but some people develop swelling of the lips or throat when they eat or drink cold foods.

Of particular concern is the fact that a cold-sensitive person may react dramatically to swimming in cold water, with a drop in blood pressure, loss of consciousness, and even drowning. There are many reasons why a person should never swim alone, and this is one more.

Allergic sensitivity to cold can start at any time of life, but it is rare and easy to self-diagnose. Hold an ice cube on your forearm for a minute or two and observe the area after removing the cube. If a hive or swelling appears a few minutes after removing the ice cube, you have developed this physical allergy.

The condition should be evaluated by a doctor to rule out underlying complications, which may include infections and blood disorders. Antihistamines, especially cyproheptadine hydrochloride (Periactin), are often effective treatment. Sometimes the condition resolves on its own.

Cholinergic urticaria. These are hives that occur when the skin is heated, whether by direct exposure to heat or hot water or through exercise or anxiety. The hives are different from most varieties, being very small and round and surrounded by redness, but they certainly itch like other hives.

Asthmalike symptoms may appear after exercise in patients with this condition, and as a result it is often confused with exercise-induced asthma. Because a hot shower can bring it on, patients sometimes speculate that they are allergic to soap or shampoo.

The treatment of choice is the antihistamine hydroxyzine hydrochloride, usually prescribed in fairly high doses.

Sensitivity to pressure on the skin. Some people have skin that is unusually sensitive to pressure. One form of this sensitivity is called dermographism, a condition in which one can write or draw on the skin. Mild pressure or scraping may quickly cause redness, swelling, and itching. If your skin is this sensitive to pressure, you are likely to develop hives in any area where clothing is tight—for example, under elastic in undergarments or around the belt line. In the delayed pressure urticaria, the hives or swelling appears usually six to eight hours after the pressure has been applied. Often these patients also have chronic idiopathic hives—i.e., the cause of the hives is unknown.

The condition should be evaluated by a doctor. Antihistamines may help. Loose clothing is certainly the dress style of choice.

Some patients have a rather serious pressure sensitivity that can cause delayed swelling and lesions in such places as the bottoms of the feet, under a bra strap, even under a wallet carried in a back pocket.

If there are incapacitating skin lesions, an oral steroid (cortisone) may be needed. As always with steroids, you want to use the lowest possible dose, preferably on alternate days. Some patients respond to nonsteroidal anti-inflammatory drugs, such as indomethacin.

Recent studies from the University of Colorado suggest that in some cases a food allergy contributes to delayed pressure sensitivity, and it does seem that occasionally patients improve after the identification of foods or additives to which they show sensitivity and the elimination of these from their diet.

Solar urticaria. This is a rare disease in which exposure to certain forms of light, in some cases sunlight, causes hives to appear within several minutes. In most cases, avoidance is the only effective treatment. One must not expose the skin to the kind of light to which one is sensitive. When sunlight is the cause of the problem, windowpanes or similar glass usually filters the light adequately for protection. Out of doors, unclothed areas of skin must be protected with sunblock.

Aquagenic urticaria. In this very rare disorder, the patient develops hives when soaked in water, regardless of the water's temperature. You must be exposed to the water for a considerable time; just washing your hands will not usually trigger the hives.

If you have this problem, do not plan to become an Olympic swimmer. Avoidance of immersion in water is the best treatment.

Hereditary vibratory urticaria. Your chance of developing this is about one in a billion, but it does illustrate the complexity of heredity and the immune system. The disease has been described in one family and in a few other sporadic cases. The hives are caused by vibration of the skin; they are not dermographic and are not induced by pressure. Avoidance of vibration is the treatment.

5. Contact with allergens. Occasionally, contact with inhalant allergens such as pollen or mold can cause urticaria. The sensitivity, called contact urticaria, can at times be confirmed by skin tests or RAST.

In one case, a woman developed chronic hives, and after a futile search for the cause a house visit revealed that she had an old-fashioned horsehair mattress. Further questioning revealed that the hives were worst in the morning and tended to fade during the day.

Sure enough, the patient was allergic to horse dander and horsehair. When she got rid of the mattress, the hives disappeared.

Hives can also result from skin contact with a chemical substance to which you are allergic, such as a dry-cleaning chemical or fabric softener. Also, contact with toxic substances or simply strong chemicals can cause skin reactions, including hives.

Diagnosis

Because urticaria does at times indicate an infection somewhere in the body, your doctor may recommend quite a few tests if you come in with a complaint of frequent or chronic hives and a cause cannot be quickly determined. A complete physical should be done. A urinalysis and blood analysis may be recommended, as well as a stool test, the purpose of which is to rule out the possibility of intestinal parasitic worms. The blood work may include a test for blood complement if angioedema is present or vasculitis is suspected. X rays of the sinuses, teeth, or chest may be ordered.

There is disagreement in the medical community as to how much testing is appropriate, and you, the consumer, should be aware of the issue. Some doctors will not advocate a comprehensive workup if your history and physical exam indicate normal health. Others take the view that some infections, such as certain sinus infections, are almost without symptoms and might be missed without X rays.

Always feel free to question the necessity for tests and to give some weight to your own common sense. Factors that certainly can be taken into consideration are how troublesome the symptom is to you and whether you generally feel well or not. The workup should be tailored to your individual situation.

Drug Treatment

In general, the best treatment for hives is avoidance of whatever triggers them. But if that is not possible, relief may be obtained in some cases from drug treatment.

In cases of acute hives, an injection of epinephrine (Adrenalin) and antihistamines, or a large oral dose of prednisone for a short period of time, can help to stop the ongoing reaction.

In rare instances, prednisone may be used to control severe outbreaks of chronic hives. But because of the serious side effects, steroids should be administered in the lowest dose possible, preferably every other day.

In most cases H1 antihistamines are the better choice for treatment of acute or chronic hives, although antihistamines do not work in all cases. The newer, nonsedating antihistamines are tolerated best by most people. Often the addition of an H2 antihistamine to the standard H1 antihistamine will improve the effectiveness of drug treatment (see chapter 5).

Causes of Angioedema

Angioedema, or swelling, frequently accompanies allergy reactions of all sorts. It is prominent in severe, acute reactions to food and drugs. It is sometimes associated with milder allergies, such as allergic rhinitis. There is even a form of angioedema that corresponds to the rare urticaria caused by vibration. Occasionally, vibration causes swelling without hives.

Angioedema should always be seen by a doctor for diagnosis. One of the goals of the evaluation of the swelling is to be certain that it is indeed allergy-related. Certain heart and kidney disorders can also cause swelling of a different sort.

Cellulitis is another condition producing swelling that may be confused with allergic angioedema. Cellulitis is something a bit more serious than the presence of so-called cellulite (fat) in the skin of the thighs and buttocks. It is an infection of the skin that requires antibiotic treatment.

Hereditary Angioedema

In the past, people suffering from this rare but severe disease were likely to die suddenly of asphyxiation. Hereditary angioedema, which typically does not appear until adolescence or later, is of autosomal dominant inheritance, which means that it will affect men and women approximately equally and will affect many members of a family. Happily, we are now able to control the disease, so it is worthwhile to get a prompt diagnosis. There is considerable risk in delaying treatment.

Basically, hereditary angioedema involves a lack of a normal blood protein, C1 esterase inhibitor. In some cases, the protein levels are too low or the protein is present but does not function. This is an evanescent substance that can only be administered intravenously.

Some of the signs of hereditary angioedema are that the angioedema is fairly long-lasting, up to several days. It can be cyclic, occurring every ten days to two weeks, or it can be quite erratic.

As a first symptom an extensive, red, burning rash may erupt. The swelling, which is not especially itchy, can take place anywhere in the body, but there is an unusual predilection for the throat and respiratory tract and the gastrointestinal tract. The condition thus causes hoarseness and choking; sometimes intense stomach pain, nausea, and vomiting occur. Frequently people with this disorder are given emergency abdominal surgery, which produces no findings.

Angioedema attacks may be triggered by soft-tissue trauma, such as dental work, oral surgery, or a tonsillectomy. Patients who have had attacks of this disease should never have surgery or dental work without first ensuring that appropriate precautions are being taken (see below).

Hereditary angioedema can be controlled by the drugs stanozolol and danazol. These are androgens related to testosterone and so must be used under a doctor's supervision to avoid unwanted side effects. C1 esterase inhibitor is not widely available. Epinephrine and antihistamine are not effective against this disease.

Before surgery or dental work, the patient can be treated with a transfusion of fresh frozen plasma, which will supply the missing C1 esterase inhibitor. Another approach, used in patients who are being treated regularly for the disease, is to raise the dose of the androgens used for a period of time before surgery.

Acquired Angioedema

When angioedema caused by C1 esterase inhibitor deficiency appears in a person who does not seem to have a family history of the disease, it is called acquired angioneurotic edema. This condition may be a feature of certain malignancies and autoimmune diseases. The treatment is to control the underlying disease, if possible.

Atopic Dermatitis and Contact Dermatitis

The second most common allergic skin disease—after urticaria, or hives—is the disease popularly known as eczema.

The term *eczema* is from ancient Greek and means "to boil over" or "to erupt." This refers to the inflammation and weeping (leaking) of the eczema rash. Actually, any inflamed, crusty, itchy rash may be called eczema, but several different conditions can produce such a rash, including atopic dermatitis, which tends to be inherited and is often associated with an allergy to some substance ingested or inhaled; and contact dermatitis, which is caused by contact with some substance to which you are sensitive or allergic, such as the resin of poison ivy. Most often, however, eczema refers to atopic dermatitis.

Atopic means "not having a place," which is an excellent description for this allergic rash, because it may appear almost anywhere on the body. It was an American pioneer in allergy, Arthur Coca, who in the early 1900s discovered that atopic dermatitis is associated with allergic rhinitis and asthma. A tendency toward developing these atopic diseases runs in families, and if you develop one, you are likely to develop another (although it is rare to have all three forms).

The itching, especially in childhood forms of the disease, is intense, and the skin lesions and related complications seem to arise primarily from scratching the affected area. The itching is often made worse by stress, sweating, irritants, and other factors, and may flare up at bedtime.

Dr. Coca and others felt that patients suffering from this disease had easily irritated nerve endings in the skin. Sometimes, therefore, the disease was called neurodermatitis. From this the public got the idea that people with atopic dermatitis are neurotic. This is not so, even though stress may aggravate the symptoms.

A well-known person who apparently suffered from atopic dermatitis exacerbated by stress was President Lyndon B. Johnson. In his recent biography of Johnson, Robert Caro describes an eczemalike rash that would develop on Johnson's hands during times of tension and unhappiness. Johnson's fingers would become dry and painful, with cracks that bled. He would not stop work but would keep a jar of lubricating lotion on his desk and wrap up his hands to protect the papers he was working with.

Incidence

Reliable figures on the incidence of atopic dermatitis are not available, but approximately 4 percent of infants and children are afflicted. The disease tends to get better in about half to two-thirds of affected infants as they get older, although adults may go on to develop irritant dermatitis—a tendency to develop rashes from exposure to dishwashing detergents, certain chemicals, and the like.

Only about 1 percent or less of adults are afflicted with atopic dermatitis, but many mild cases probably are not reported. A tendency to dry skin may be the only lingering sign of the disease. When skin is more than normally dry—say, as a result of low humidity or frequent washing with soap and hot water—the skin may become uncomfortable or a rash may flare up. A mild tendency to rashes may be aggravated by working in wet conditions or occupations in which one must wash one's hands frequently; water tends to dry the skin by removing natural oils.

Almost all cases of the disease begin before age five, two-thirds arising under age one. In infants, the face is typically affected first, along with the lower abdomen. A few months later, a rash is likely to appear on the legs and forearms. In older children and adults, the insides of the elbows and backs of the knees are the most common sites. The backs of the hands and feet are also frequently affected. One sees more boys than girls with atopic dermatitis in early childhood. This reverses as children get older.

The rash is typically in the form of red patches, followed by thickening and scaling of the skin, with the affected areas becoming a darker red. In infants and in children aged up to three or four, the rash is likely to weep (leak fluid). Thereafter, weeping may stop, but the disease may cause a thickening of the skin (lichenification).

Physiological Mechanisms

Medical researchers are still working to discover the exact mechanisms underlying flare-ups of atopic dermatitis. Numerous studies indicate that the immune system in these patients is abnormal in several subtle ways. There may be abnormal lymphocytes, and mast cells that infiltrate the skin of such patients.

Also, the blood flow to the skin is abnormal, leading to a condition called white dermographism. Dermographism is the tendency for the skin to develop red streaks under even slight pressure. (These streaks may swell and develop as hives.) In atopic dermatitis, when you rub the skin, red streaks appear, but then they quickly turn whitish, and this white dermographism persists for several minutes.

About 80 percent of people with atopic dermatitis have very high levels of the allergy antibody IgE in their blood and decreased levels of the important chemical substance CAMP in their white blood cells (see chapter 9).

Many atopic dermatitis patients show an unusual number of positive results when given skin tests for allergies. Frequently these results have no clinical significance—they are unrelated to the disease. In some patients, however, allergic sensitivity is linked to flare-ups of the rash.

Food allergy has long been recognized as a cause of some cases of atopic dermatitis. In addition, recent research by Drs. Alan Adinoff and Richard Clark at the National Jewish Center for Immunology and Respiratory Medicine in Denver, Colorado, suggests that an allergic sensitivity to environmental allergens, such as pollen, dust mites, and dander, also may cause a rash to flare up.

The immune mechanism underlying this kind of dermatitis is not well understood, but it is known that the mechanism is not the same as the standard mast cell–mediated reaction that governs most allergies.

Finally, atopic-dermatitis patients have impaired cellular immunity, with a susceptibility to developing viral and bacterial skin infections. If you are prone to this kind of dermatitis, you should be aware of the risk, and get to a doctor promptly if a rash is more severe or more persistent than usual.

If the rash is weeping, crusted, or has small pustules (white bumps), it should be checked by a doctor. Also, a doctor should look at any rash that lasts more than a week. Staphylococcus bacteria are common infectious agents. The next most likely villain is the streptococcus type of bacteria. Antibiotic treatment is required to clear up these infections.

Viral infections can be more complicated to treat. For instance, infection by herpes simplex (eczema herpeticum) was once very difficult to treat; there were potentially fatal complications. Oral acyclovir now is used to control the herpes. But a doctor should supervise the care of the rash.

Other complications of atopic dermatitis that require expert medical care are nipple lesions and involvement of the eyes. Patients are also prone to develop cataracts (even early in life), abrasions and infections (especially by a type of herpes virus) of the cornea, retinal detachment, and harmful rashes on the eyelids.

Eating citrus fruit may cause lesions around the mouth and occasionally even furrows on the lips.

Diagnosis of Atopic Dermatitis

There is no single test or sign by which to identify atopic dermatitis. A doctor will look for the following characteristics. Three are considered adequate to make the diagnosis.

- The rash is itchy.
- The rash begins as red patches; these thicken and darken, and the skin scales. In infants, particularly, the rash may weep (leak fluid).
- The rash follows a typical distribution for the age of the patient.

- The rash tends to be chronic. It repeatedly flares up or follows a seasonal pattern, worsening in winter, when the air is dry.
- The patient or the patient's family has a history of atopic diseases (allergic rhinitis, asthma, and atopic dermatitis).

The presence of three or more of the following features will tend to confirm the diagnosis:

- Positive results in skin testing for allergens such as pollen and dander.
- Elevated levels of the allergy antibody IgE.
- A tendency to develop skin infections.
- Lesions of the nipple.
- In the eye, a distortion of the cornea (keratoconus) and a certain type of cataract.
- Itchiness when sweating.
- Intolerance of wool on the skin.
- Intolerance of certain foods.
- White dermographism.
- Exacerbation by stress or other emotional factors or by environmental factors, such as chemical fumes in the workplace.

An eczemalike rash that is sometimes misdiagnosed as atopic dermatitis is caused by scabies. This disease, produced by a skin infestation of tiny scabies mites, is extremely itchy and can seriously undermine the patient's health. A clue to the diagnosis may be given in the location of the rash, as scabies prefer certain tender areas of the skin: wrists and armpits; between the fingers; the groin; and toes. In infants, they often go for the scalp, face, palms, and soles of the feet. Confirmation of the diagnosis is by microscopic examination of a small skin sample.

Psoriasis, a nonallergic disease involving excess production of skin cells, causes a much scalier rash and sometimes joint pain and swelling. It tends to affect the arms, scalp, ears, and groin.

Allergy Tests

Food allergies in about 10 percent of patients are associated with flare-ups of atopic dermatitis. Therefore, avoidance of problem foods can be helpful, even though food is rarely the sole cause of atopic dermatitis.

The foods associated with the rash can usually be identified through the history that you give your doctor, but sometimes an elimination diet or challenge testing is needed to detect the food or foods to which you are sensitive (see chapter 7). The most common problem foods are eggs, cow's milk, soy, wheat, peanuts, and fish.

If avoidance of a given food helps to clear up the rashes, part of your problem is probably solved. But no one, especially a child, should be kept for long on a restricted diet without double-checking that the apparent allergy really is present. If you have never shown any violent reaction to the suspect food, you may simply try some from time to time to see if it still causes flare-ups of dermatitis; but discuss this with your doctor.

If your food sensitivity has ever caused a severe reaction, with swelling or other systemic symptoms, then of course you should not experiment on your own. But an allergist, using care, can run a challenge test with small amounts of the suspect food to verify the diagnosis.

Accurate testing is not easy (see chapter 7). How best to test becomes even more complicated with atopic-dermatitis patients, because their skin is often highly reactive to any stimulus. This makes reliable skin tests, both for food and for inhalant allergens, more difficult to accomplish. In these patients, skin testing may yield more false positives than is normally the case. However, skin testing can be performed if the doctor finds the negative control is not any more reactive than normal skin and the doctor can find areas of normal skin to work with.

In the experience of the authors, in vitro tests (RAST) are more helpful in any case with significant skin disease, but these tests also yield false positive results. Therefore, some doctors prefer to start with skin tests, running a preliminary test with a control substance to find an area of skin that is not overreactive.

Both in vivo and in vitro tests are more reliable in children, and the positive tests have much greater validity. But *negative* RAST or skin tests in both children and adults are helpful in that they rule out an allergy to that food. What kind of tests to run and in what sequence and combination are questions about which capable, well-trained allergists still frequently disagree. As always, not too much reliance should be put on any one test.

Treatment

The treatment of atopic dermatitis associated with inhalant allergens (dust mites, dander, pollen, or the like) is by avoidance of the allergens, in combination with treatment of the rash itself.

Unless the patient also has other allergic conditions, such as rhinitis or asthma, it is not a good idea to treat atopic-dermatitis patients with allergy shots because they are not effective. Generally, treatment of atopic dermatitis, when it is chronic, requires a variety of approaches. An allergist will often work with a dermatologist on treatment.

People with atopic dermatitis have extremely dry skin because water does not bind properly in the skin and is rapidly lost. Thus, replacing water is the key to therapy in any stage of the illness. The patient should take a soaking bath or shower in tepid water for 20 minutes at least twice a day. Pat the skin dry (do not rub) and then apply an emollient (Alpha Keri, Carmol, Keri, Lubriderm) to prevent water from evaporating from the skin.

Topical steroids may be prescribed, and the time to apply them is within several minutes of bathing, because they penetrate better when the skin is moist. Apply the steroids first and then an emollient in other places where the steroids are not needed. In severe cases, wet wraps may be used after bathing.

Hot water should be avoided. Bath oils do not help the dermatitis, and they also make the tub slippery, increasing the possibility of an accident. The addition of oatmeal (Aveeno) to the bath, however, can be soothing. The best choice of soap may require a little experimenting.

For wet, weepy lesions, your doctor may suggest compresses with Burow's 1:40 solution or one packet of Domeboro powder per quart of water. Such a compress works as an astringent and antibacterial agent. But these compresses should not be used for more than two or three days, because they can be drying.

Infection, of course, is a constant concern, and may require antibiotic therapy. This should be under the supervision of a physician. Only oral antibiotics can be used. Neither over-the-counter nor prescription antibiotic creams or ointments are helpful.

Topical steroids, which are the mainstay of pharmaceutical treatment, must be used with caution because of their side effects. The guiding principle is to use the weakest concentration that will work.

The most potent topical steroids cause thinning of the skin and cannot be used daily over long periods of time. The potency of the steroid is related to the degree of fluorination (which makes the steroid molecules stronger) and to the amount of the steroid in the cream or ointment.

Except under the direction of a dermatologist, do not use anything stronger than 1 percent hydrocortisone cream or ointment on the face, neck, or any body fold area, such as the groin or armpit. These areas have the thinnest layer of skin, and are very vulnerable to atrophy.

Incidentally, the choice of whether to use a cream or ointment is best made by your doctor. Ointments decrease water loss but may increase itchiness. Creams spread more easily but may cause drying.

A medium-strength steroid preparation is ordinarily the drug of choice. Very potent steroids have to be used with great caution. One sound approach is use of the strongest steroids in the early, severe stages of the rash, switching to weaker concentrations as the condition improves.

Over-the-counter cortisone preparations typically come in 0.5 percent strength. You may be able to use these to treat very mild rashes yourself, but if the problem persists for more than a week or two, you really should see a doctor.

Another type of topical treatment is the application of tar-based ointments, such as Estar Gel. These help some patients. Others find them irritating and the odor unpleasant. Sometimes it is helpful to use them at bedtime and then wash them off in the morning bath or shower, so that you do not carry the odor all day.

Some people report partial relief from antihistamines, but that may be because the sedating effect reduces the intense itching. Curiously, high doses of aspirin may also calm the itching in some patients, but aspirin must be administered under the guidance of a doctor because of the side effects of large doses.

Sunlight helps to clear some cases of atopic dermatitis, but the patient must avoid sunburn, high humidity, and getting too warm, which can worsen the rash. Sun-lamp treatment helps in some cases, but it should be done only under the guidance of a physician.

Most people with atopic dermatitis find that they have to avoid certain substances and activities that irritate the skin. Soap and detergents, cleaning solvents, wool and nylon clothing, plastic covers on bedding can all cause flare-ups of the rash.

Frequent washing with hot water is apt to cause a reaction, as will sweating, in patients with severe dermatitis. Exposure to hot, dusty environments, to animals, and to many chemicals may exacerbate the disease.

Some doctors recommend not washing in water and using antiseptic lotions instead. But as a rule, it seems more effective to bathe and clean the skin well, using a hypoallergenic or lubricating soap and a hypoallergenic moisturizer to prevent drying.

Contact Dermatitis

Rashes caused by contact with irritants or with substances to which you are allergic are called contact dermatitis. Technically, allergists are concerned only with allergic contact dermatitis (ACD), not irritant contact dermatitis. But since the exact cause and nature of the dermatitis often cannot be quickly determined—and since the patients want relief whatever the cause—allergists and dermatologists typically treat both sorts of rashes. What is important is that these specialists consult in difficult cases.

Actually, a number of substances, such as cement and industrial chemicals, can act as both allergic agents and irritants, and irritant dermatitis is often a complication of some other skin disease, such as atopic dermatitis or psoriasis. Patients with atopic dermatitis are at increased risk for contact dermatitis and should avoid topical antihistamines, antibiotics, and anesthetics, which frequently cause contact dermatitis.

ACD does not arise on first exposure to a substance but only after you have already become sensitized to it. But exposure to one substance to which you build up a sensitivity may also give rise to an allergy to a related substance.

The physiology of this type of allergy response depends on the sensitization of certain white blood cells—T cell lymphocytes—to particular substances that are then recognized as antigens when they enter the body. When a T cell meets a molecule of an antigen, it produces substances called lymphokines. Among the functions of the lymphokines is attracting big, hungry macrophages to the region; these are white blood cells that specialize in gobbling up and destroying foreign substances in your body, whether they be bacteria or otherwise harmless molecules of poison-ivy antigen.

Incidentally, one of the lymphokines is interferon, a substance that is being used widely to fight a number of diseases.

The response that underlies ACD does not involve the allergy antibody, IgE, but it is an immune-system response. It is also called a cell-mediated response or delayed hypersensitivity, the latter because it takes about two days to develop.

Poison Ivy

Poison ivy is a good example of an ACD itchy rash. Also, if you have become sensitized to any member of this plant family (poison ivy, poison oak, and poison sumac), you are likely to be sensitive to all members.

When they have been pulled up, these plants should be buried or else discarded in the wild. Burning them creates dangerous fumes.

If you live in poison-ivy country, it is best to police your property fairly regularly so that the vines do not proliferate. They are quite difficult to kill off once they are well established, and for some people even slight contact will provoke a rash.

Treating Poison Ivy

If you are sensitive to poison ivy, poison oak, or poison sumac, there is a new, nonprescription topical cream containing TEA stearate and stearate MEA, called Ivy Shield, that you can apply before exposure to reduce the severity of a reaction by up to 50 percent. Of course, avoiding these plants is best, but if you want to hike or camp out, complete avoidance may be difficult.

Researchers are currently studying whether organo clay may

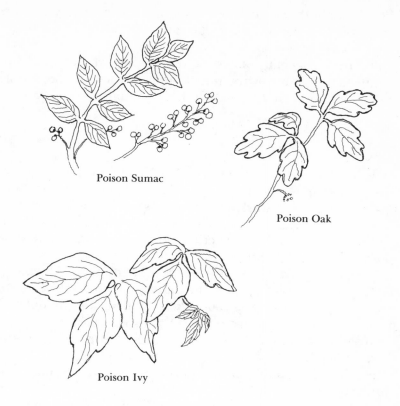

Poison Sumac

Poison Oak

Poison Ivy

provide an even more effective shield. This substance is used as a filler in deodorant, but do not try to use deodorant as a shield. The filler is not present in large enough quantities to help against poison ivy.

The sensitizing substance in poison ivy and its cousins is an oil, uroshiol, that sticks to all surfaces. Isopropyl alcohol, which tends to deactivate it, can be applied to skin, clothing, and work tools as needed. Washing down with alcohol or plain water after exposure may help, but soap may spread the oil on your skin. The oil may also be spread if you take a hot bath.

Pets can carry the poison-ivy oil, and children who hug and kiss dogs, baby goats, and other lovable animals may develop whopping cases of poison ivy. A child or anyone with a dramatic case of poison ivy should be seen by a doctor, especially if there is swelling, as of the hands or lips, or if large areas of skin are affected.

For mild outbreaks of poison ivy, over-the-counter cortisone ointments are probably the best treatment. Calamine lotion and other drying agents should not be used.

There is a possibility of desensitization through shots and oral immunization, but this treatment approach has not been fully studied yet and is not recommended. Avoidance is still best.

Other Causes of ACD

ACD is a fairly common industrial complaint, and in some industrial factories as much as 10 percent of the work force has this disease. If your work environment seems to cause rashes or hives in a significant number of those who are on site, you should probably try to find out whether the situation also may pose more serious health risks.

ACD affects older people more frequently than the young. To take an example of one of the most common sensitivities, 14 percent of women over age 50 are allergic to nickel, but only 2.2 percent of girls under age ten react to nickel. This is evidently because in most, though not all, cases of ACD it takes months or years of exposure to develop the sensitivity.

In some cases, sunlight breaks down a substance that ordinarily causes no problem into components that may produce a reaction. This is photo-contact dermatitis. For instance you may wear a perfume on your body with no problem until one day you splash a little on your neck and temples before going out to watch a tennis tournament. Later a rash appears on your face.

Symptoms

The ACD rash often begins as redness of the skin, with bumps and blistering following. It usually appears within a few days after contact with the offending substance. Typically, the edge of the rash is sharp, or clearly defined, which is a clue to the diagnosis. The rash itches, and if it is situated near the eyes, swelling resembling angioedema may occur. In chronic forms of the disease, there is less blistering and more crusting and scaling.

The rash is most likely to appear on the neck, eyelids, and groin. Perspiration and rubbing will make the skin more susceptible to the rash.

Diagnosis of ACD

The basic evidence for the diagnosis is the history of the circumstances in which the rash erupts and the clinical appearance of the rash: Is it well demarcated? Are there small blisters? In addition, patch testing can be done to confirm a diagnosis.

In patch testing, an adhesive patch with a suspect substance is applied to the skin. The patch is left in place for 48 hours, then removed, and the skin is examined for a reaction. The area should be checked again in a day or two, and then again a week later, to see if there is a late reaction.

If you start to itch intensely before the 48 hours are up, call your doctor. The patch should probably be taken off early.

Often several patches are applied at once; but one drawback to patch testing is that your skin may become "excited" and react to a number of substances whether you are allergic to them or not. Therefore, if there are multiple positive tests, it is often advisable to retest a suspect substance alone at a later date to be sure that the test result was accurate.

Accuracy of the patch tests is improved by avoiding vigorous physical activity and baths during the time the patch is in place.

Rare side effects of patch testing include anaphylactic reactions. These occur within minutes after contact. Also, again rarely, the test procedure may sensitize the patient to the substance being tested.

There are countless substances that may cause ACD, so random testing may be useless as well as quite expensive. But there is a screening set of tests for 20 substances most often implicated in ACD. These are chemicals and drugs commonly encountered in cosmetics, in cleaning fluids, as local anesthetics, in hobby shops, and so on. They are benzocaine, 2-mercaptobenzothiazole, colophony, p-phenylenediamine, imidazolidinyl urea, cinnamic aldehyde, lanolin alcohol, Carba rubber mix, neomycin, formaldehyde, thiuram rubber mix, ethylenediamine, epoxy resin, mercapto rubber mix, black rubber mix, butylphenol formaldehyde resin, potassium dichromate, quaternium 15, balsam of Peru, and nickel sulfate.

The place on the body that the rash appears often gives clues as to the possible cause. A general body rash is likely to be caused by resins, dyes, formaldehyde in synthetic fabrics, or rubber in garments. The following table gives the most likely causes of rashes that are confined to various sites:

Allergies

Area	Cause
Feet	Shoes, foot-care products, shower sandals, medication for athlete's foot
Genitals, male	Jock-itch medication, condoms, vaginal medications or contraceptive medication used by sexual partner
Genitals, female	Contraceptive medication, rubber diaphragm, scented sanitary pads, deodorants, douches, condoms
Anal region	Hemorrhoid medication
Hands	Hand-care medicines and lotions, rubber gloves, metal jewelry, plants
Underarm region	Deodorants, fabric or rubber in garments, perfume
Forehead, neck, and shoulders	Hair dyes, hair-care products, cosmetics, sunscreens, topical medicines, perfumes, nickel in jewelry, garments, hatbands
Ears	Nickel in earrings, perfumes, earplugs, earphones, and the like
Eyelids	Cosmetics, eye drops, nail polish, hair spray and other hair products, chemical fumes such as those from epoxy resins
Lips	Lipstick, lip protectors, toothpaste, mouthwash, fruits or other food, rubber erasers
Face in general	Cosmetics, topical medications, plants, shaving aids, fumes such as those from epoxy resins, sunscreens

The history that you give the doctor should cover occupation, hobbies, and habits. Sometimes a normally benign item, such as a nibbled-upon pencil eraser, turns out to be the culprit.

A savvy physician, however, will hope to find the cause quickly by focusing on the following questions:

• Do you wear jewelry containing nickel?
• Do you work with cement or in the tanning, dyeing, or printing industries? The common ingredient that causes trouble in all these occupations is chromium salt. Other elements and chemical compounds used in these industries may also cause skin reactions.
• Do you work with or frequently handle plants?
• What cosmetics and hair products do you use?
• What perfumes and deodorants do you use? (There are so many substances present in cosmetics, hair products, perfumes, body lotions, and so on that you may have to write the company that makes the product for a complete list of ingredients.)

• Do you have pets? (They can carry resin from poison ivy on their coats.)

• Are you using any topical medications, such as an antibiotic cream, local anesthetic or anti-inflammatory ointment, eye-drops, antibacterial agents? Be aware that it may not be the main ingredient but a preservative—for example, parabens—that is the problem.

• Are you frequently in contact with soaps, detergents, bleaches, furniture oils, paint and paint thinner, and other common cleaning and painting products? Do you rinse clothes thoroughly to remove cleaning agents?

• Are you exposed to formaldehyde in your work, clothing, or environment? Health-care and lab workers formerly were widely exposed to formaldehyde used as a preservative. Since it is now recognized as a carcinogen, it is used less. But it is also present in some common products, including certain kinds of wallboard and newly purchased permanent-press clothing. With wallboard, the formaldehyde is supposed to be subject to treatment that fixes it in the board. Reportedly, defective wallboard is sometimes installed.

Treatment

In acute contact dermatitis, with an extensive rash, cold wet dressings with dilute Burow's solution may be recommended.

In later stages of the rash topical steroids are very effective, but be sure to follow the safety precautions outlined in the discussion of atopic dermatitis, above. You must follow the prescription directions, and never use a strong topical steroid cream or ointment on your face or other parts of the body where the skin is thin.

Oral steroids may be needed for a short period. Antihistamines may relieve the itching. If an infection superimposed on the rash threatens, your doctor may prescribe oral antibiotics.

If you have sensitive skin—if, for example, you already suffer from atopic dermatitis—you should avoid coming in contact with substances that tend to produce irritations. Some topical drugs very frequently cause sensitization and should be avoided. These include topical antihistamines, antibiotics, and benzocaine and other local anesthetics.

One patient being treated for nasal allergies and atopic dermatitis (primarily by allergy shots) responded well for several years, but then developed an eczemalike rash on her hands, eyelids, and to a small extent on her face. One approach would be to stop using all cosmetics, perfumes, face creams and so on, but who wants to live that way? Finally—after a lot of work— her doctor isolated the problem. She had an unusual contact allergy to sorbic acid, which was in a perfume that she used.

Armed with a list of things that contain sorbic acid, she avoided trouble. But one day she had an EKG and, eight hours later, there was dermatitis on every spot where the electrodes had been placed. She had told the technician of her allergies, including the sensitivity to sorbic acid, but he had not thoroughly checked the label on the EKG jelly. This illustrates an important point: if you have allergies, it is always risky to take anyone else's word for the ingredients in anything. Luckily, no real harm was done.

13

Anaphylaxis

It is extremely important to be alert to the possibility that an allergic reaction may take the form of anaphylaxis, that is, a rapidly developing systemic allergic reaction that can lead to shock and even death. The silver lining is that the total number of deaths from anaphylaxis is relatively low, approximately 1 for every 2.5 million people per year.

Among the most common causes of anaphylaxis discussed so far are allergies to peanuts and penicillin. There is also the rare danger of an allergy-immunization treatment causing anaphylaxis. Many impatient patients feel that their doctors are being overcautious when they insist on the half-hour waiting period in the office after an allergy shot. But even when treated, anaphylaxis has a mortality rate of up to 10 percent, so a responsible doctor will not want to allow the slightest risk of a patient going into anaphylaxis without medical attention at hand.

Anaphylaxis can be induced not only by certain food and drug allergies but also by hypersensitivity to insect stings, which is the most common cause, accounting for some 40 deaths annually in the United States. Serious, nonfatal reactions to stings occur in approximately 1 person per 20,000 each year.

Under some circumstances, anaphylaxis can be brought on by a reaction to vigorous exercise. There is also a form of anaphylaxis called idiopathic, which means that we don't know what causes it.

Anaphylaxis has been recognized as a syndrome since ancient times, but it is only in the past 100 years that we have developed an understanding of the physiology of the reaction. In 1900 Charles Richet and Paul Portier undertook research that ultimately clarified the cause of many mysterious deaths.

Richet and Portier studied the toxic qualities of the tentacles of the Portuguese man-of-war. They injected dogs with different amounts of the toxin to determine fatal levels and to see whether one could build up an immunity or tolerance to the toxin. To their surprise, dogs receiving a second injection at very low, presumably almost harmless, dosage levels suddenly died. Richet and Portier called this result anaphylactic, meaning "contrary to protection." They were contrasting it to the prophylactic, or protective, effect that they had expected.

In this same period, other researchers discovered that anaphylaxis could be caused by nontoxic proteins, including animal blood serum. Richet went on to theorize that some special substance in the blood of sensitized animals must react with the toxin to produce the anaphylactic disorder. He was on the right track, and in 1913 his work was recognized with a Nobel Prize.

Until the post–World War II era, horse serum, used in various immunizations and treatments for infection, was a leading cause of anaphylaxis. Tetanus treatment and prophylaxis, in particular, was done widely with horse serum and caused severe reactions once in a while.

Today human serum is available for tetanus treatment, and it is preferred. But in the meantime, penicillin has become one of the most widely administered drugs in the world—and one of the most common causes of anaphylaxis.

Occasionally a patient will have a severe allergic reaction to a muscle relaxant or other drug used in general anesthesia. This is scary, because the patient is already asleep and the reaction is somewhat difficult to spot, unless it shows up clearly in the skin—with hives, for example. But an alert anesthesiologist will note a change in the patient's blood pressure or breathing status, indications that the patient is in trouble, and quick action can be taken. Anaphylaxis occurs in 1 of 15,000 instances of anesthesia, but only 3 percent of anaphylactic reactions during surgery result in death.

The possibility of an allergic reaction is one of the many reasons to be very conservative in using general anesthesia—but most people would heartily agree that it is not a reason to forgo necessary treatment that requires a general anesthetic.

Characteristics of Anaphylaxis

That special substance in the blood that Richet hypothesized must react with the toxin is, we now know, the allergy antibody IgE. True anaphylactic reactions result from the action of IgE on the mast cells in connective tissue and the basophils in blood, which release chemical mediators that cause allergy symptoms.

Some purists use the term *anaphylaxis* to refer to any IgE-mediated allergy reaction, but most often the term is reserved for the rapid and overwhelming reaction that involves numerous organs and can lead to death within minutes.

A similar process not involving IgE is called anaphylactoid, meaning "like anaphylaxis." One of the most common causes of anaphylactoid reactions is the use of radiographic contrast substances in taking X rays. Some people are sensitive to these dyes, and no sooner is the contrast medium injected than the patient reacts with symptoms of anaphylaxis, such as hives, angioedema (swelling), and, in very serious cases, swelling of the trachea and/or shock. Since this ordinarily happens in a hospital setting, the patient usually can be brought around quickly with injections of epinephrine, antihistamines, and steroids. Otherwise, the mortality rate might be high indeed.

Another cause of anaphylactoid reactions is sensitivity to aspirin and other nonsteroidal anti-inflammatory drugs.

The distinction between anaphylactic and anaphylactoid reactions is of no great importance to the patient, but in theory the former requires some prior exposure to the reaction-causing substance, whereas an anaphylactoid reaction can occur—and often does occur—on the first exposure.

There have been isolated reports of IgE-mediated anaphylaxis seeming to occur upon first exposure, but most likely the patient was exposed to the substance or a related substance earlier without realizing it.

The symptoms of anaphylaxis are unforgettable to anyone who has been through them. They typically begin to appear within seconds to about 15 minutes after exposure. In response to the histamine and other chemical mediators that are flooding into the body, capillaries open, the bronchial tubes constrict, and there is excess mucus production and swelling (edema), sometimes accompanied by hives and itching. Swelling of the throat and larynx, which causes hoarseness, choking, and difficulty swallowing, is particularly dangerous. It may first be felt as a lump in the throat or, if the reaction is to food, as a numbness or tingling in the mouth. The skin flushes. Blood pressure drops. The patient feels light-headed, faint, breathless, and sometimes nauseated and sick all over. Cramps and diarrhea may ensue. The patient may have increasing difficulty breathing, the skin may take on a cyanotic (bluish) tinge—indicating oxygen deprivation—and the heartbeat may become irregular. The patient may feel anxious and sense impending doom.

Occasionally, an anaphylactic reaction may be delayed for an hour or several hours. Such reactions are usually less severe.

Most deaths occur among adults, and it seems that risk of anaphylaxis increases somewhat with age. Heightened sensitivity because of repeated exposure to allergens, plus generally weaker health, accounts for the greater risk as time goes on.

People with other allergic illnesses (rhinitis, eczema, or asthma) do not as a rule seem to be any more likely to develop anaphylaxis, although among asthmatics the reaction may be more severe. For example, people with asthma may suffer slightly worse anaphylaxis from a reaction to penicillin and certain other drugs, even though their risk of reacting is the same as that of the population in general. But in the case of anaphylactoid reactions to radiographic contrast media, the presence of another allergy may predispose you slightly to the reaction.

Occupation and location may also put you at greater risk for anaphylaxis. For example, beekeepers lead dangerous lives. If you come from the South and have fire ants in your backyard, you are more at risk than a native of Alaska. Repeated exposure to a certain substance can trigger an anaphylactic attack. People having kidney dialysis treatments sometimes become sensitive to ethylene oxide gas, used to sterilize surgical instruments.

The following substances are among those reported to have caused anaphylactic or anaphylactoid reactions:

Antibiotics. Penicillin, cephalosporins, tetracycline, nitrofurantoin, streptomycin (see chapter 8 on drug allergies).
Local anesthetics. There are more than 100 kinds.

Anti-inflammatories. Aspirin, ibuprofen, indomethacin, fenoprofen, naproxen, tolmetin.

Enzymes. Chymopapain (used to treat herniated spinal disks), chymotrypsin (used to treat digestive problems), streptokinase (used to dissolve clotted blood and thus a treatment for heart attacks).

Psyllium. Present in laxatives and added to cereals.

Hormones and serums. Insulin, ACTH (adreno-corticotropic hormone), parathyroid, cortisone, horse antibody (horse serum).

Diagnostic agents. Iodinated contrast media and dyes, such as Bromsulphalein (BSP), which is used in liver testing.

Food. Peanuts and other legumes, eggs, fish and shellfish, milk, and tree nuts. Less commonly, grains, seeds, and fruits may cause an anaphylactic reaction in someone who is sensitive to the particular food (see chapter 7).

Health-food stores carry "bee pollen" (mostly dandelion pollen), as well as sunflower seeds and chamomile tea, all of which can occasionally cause a systemic reaction in hypersensitive persons, who are often also sensitive to ragweed pollen. Sulfites used to preserve food and drinks may also cause anaphylaxis.

Anaphylaxis can occur during the transfusion of blood or blood products. This can be the result of antigens in the donor's blood to which the patient is sensitive, such as egg protein. The reaction is more apt to occur among people who lack one of the immunoglobulins, IgA.

A drug called protamine sulfate, which is derived from fish sperm, is used to counteract overdoses of the blood thinner heparin; it can cause anaphylaxis in people allergic to fish. Men who are infertile or who have had a vasectomy are more commonly allergic to protamine.

Seminal fluid evidently can cause an anaphylactic reaction in a woman. A few cases have been reported. The only protection seems to be for the man to use a condom.

Exercise-induced and Idiopathic Anaphylaxis

As noted previously, *idiopathic* means "of unknown cause." It is appropriate to link idiopathic anaphylaxis with exercise-induced anaphylaxis, since the latter is quite mysterious, too.

Anaphylaxis after vigorous exercise is rare but well documented. It is sometimes associated with eating prior to exercise or with eating certain foods (such as celery or shellfish) before exercise. Probably, if you have ever had an anaphylactic attack associated with exercise and eating, you should not eat anything for two to four hours before exercise, and some doctors would advise leaving a 12-hour period.

Many patients who have experienced exercise-induced anaphylaxis also have one of the atopic allergic diseases (asthma, rhinitis, eczema), and even more have relatives with these diseases.

Some women experience the reaction only during certain phases of their menstrual cycle.

If you develop hives or itching while exercising, stop at once. If you have had an anaphylactic reaction while exercising, carry emergency medication—injectable epinephrine (Adrenalin)—and never exercise alone.

If you have had one or more anaphylactic reactions for no known reason, you, too, should carry Adrenalin.

A typical case of idiopathic anaphylaxis is that of a healthy woman, age 35, in New York City, who on a normal afternoon was speaking on the phone with her stepson, who lived about 20 blocks away. He began to realize that she seemed to be ill and fading, and then she hung up. He called 911, found a taxi, and arrived to find her unconscious with the paramedics working on her. (Her embarrassed husband, who'd been working in a home office, hadn't heard a thing until the medics banged on the door.)

The diagnosis at the hospital was anaphylaxis, but no cause was found. In three years, the incident did not recur, but following the advice of her doctor, the woman carries epinephrine (Adrenalin) and a card in her wallet identifying her problem.

In repeated cases, ongoing doses of antihistamines and even ongoing, alternate-day cortisone are used to try to stop the recurrences.

In any case of idiopathic anaphylaxis, it is important to be certain that the cause is not a sensitivity to sulfites, used as a preservative in many foods, or to a food itself. Wine contains sulfites and is a notorious cause of sulfite reactions.

Insect Stings

Insects, which are far more numerous than *Homo sapiens* and probably better adapted for survival, add injury to insult by stinging and biting us whenever possible (or so it sometimes seems). The stings can cause anaphylactic and toxic reactions, with about 0.5 percent of the population believed to be susceptible to anaphylaxis following a sting. Insects also carry diseases, from tetanus to malaria.

If you get a bee sting, you should get a tetanus booster if it has been more than ten years since your last shot. If you cannot get the booster within 24 hours, then discuss with a physician what precautions you might take. The incidence of tetanus is low, but the death rate following a tetanus infection is high.

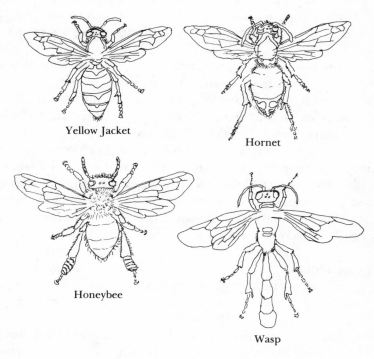

Yellow Jacket

Hornet

Honeybee

Wasp

Common Stinging Insects

There are three major families of stinging insects in the hymenoptera order: apids (bees), vespids (wasps), and formicids (ants). The apid family includes honeybees and bumblebees (which are mild-mannered). The vespid family includes hornets and yellow jackets, as well as wasps. The members of the formicid family that concern us most here are fire ants, which are found mostly in the South. Harvester ants, a mere quarter-inch in size, also sting (they can paralyze and kill small animals) and can cause anaphylaxis. They live primarily in desert areas of the western and southwestern United States.

Rarely but occasionally, other bugs also cause systemic reactions. These lesser bad guys include kissing bugs (found in southwestern states), deer flies, and bedbugs.

The venom stinging insects inject into their victims is composed of enzymes, amines, and proteins. The exact mix varies from species to species, but related insects may carry types of venom similar enough to cause cross-sensitivity. Thus, if you are allergic to one member of the vespid family, you may be allergic to others. This is particularly true of yellow jackets and hornets.

Various components of insect venom are allergenic, but the most important allergens are the enzymes phospholipase and hyaluronidase.

Insect venom can be sufficiently strong to cause serious toxic reactions even in people who are not allergic. Sometimes the typical local reaction of swelling and redness can become alarmingly more extensive. For example, a hornet sting on the hand will ordinarily result in swelling and soreness in the hand. But if the arm, too, swells up, that can be a matter of concern. Multiple stings can put a person in mortal danger, with or without an allergy reaction. About 0.5 percent of the population is believed to be susceptible to developing anaphylaxis following a sting. About 40 persons die in the United States each year from allergic reactions to stings.

Honeybees (and only honeybees, not vespids) leave their stingers and venom sacs behind. As quickly as possible after a bee sting, flick away the stinger with a fingernail or knife blade. Do not pluck out the stinger with your fingers or tweezers, as this may just squeeze more venom into the puncture.

Application of ice packs or cold soaks will retard the spread of the venom. Meat tenderizer tends to neutralize the venom and limit the local reaction but not a systemic reaction.

If you know that you are allergic, and you have Adrenalin, use it immediately after being stung by an insect. Call 911 or an ambulance service or your doctor for further help, as advised above. Apply ice. You may also use a tourniquet above the sting, but it is very important to loosen the tourniquet for one minute every three minutes.

To illustrate how quickly one must sometimes take action, consider the case of a pharmacist from Los Angeles who was traveling to a convention in the South about 12 years ago. He was alone in his car when a yellow jacket made a direct hit on his face. He winced, but there was no awful pain and so he kept driving. About five minutes later, he became aware of tightness in his chest, he felt hot, and his face had puffed to about twice its normal size.

He considered pulling over to the side of the road but realized that he had to try to get to the nearest hospital, which he estimated to be about five minutes away. He kept driving fast and held his hand hard on the horn. Luckily a state trooper saw him and pulled him over, and even more luckily the officer recognized the emergency and in about two minutes delivered him to the hospital, where he received epinephrine and steroids, antihistamines, intravenous replacement of fluid, and oxygen.

After a serious sting and anaphylactic reaction, your body is depleted of IgE and probably you will not have another major allergic reaction for several weeks, even if stung again. Don't bet your life on this—individuals do vary—but you should be aware of the possibility of IgE depletion, because if you are tested for venom sensitivity in this period, the results may be negative. The tests should not be run until a month or more after the episode. In the meantime, do see an allergist and get instruction on how to use Adrenalin.

Unfortunately, delayed reactions to stings can lead to such serious problems as kidney disease, vascular disease, fever and serum sickness, neuritis, and arthritislike symptoms.

If you have been stung and have had a reaction, try to collect or have someone else collect the carcass of the bug or one of its companions. Doctors often prefer to identify the bug themselves, for many people have difficulty distinguishing between yellow jackets and hornets, for example, or even honeybees and yellow jackets. If immunization is to be done once you have recovered, then it will help to know which creature stung you, even though you will be tested for a sensitivity to the venom of all or most species.

Big fat bumblebees are easy to identify. Honeybees are small, usually yellow or brownish, and chunky, with a round thorax (the part of the body near the head).

Vespids are recognizable by their narrow waists between thorax and abdomen. Yellow jackets have rather handsome bands of yellow and black, and are relatively svelte in build. They are the insects most often seen buzzing around garbage bins in picnic areas. They love sweets.

Hornets usually have white or yellow stripes and a white face. Their large, conical, gray or tan nests are typically located at a considerable height, in a tree or under eaves, for example.

Yellow jackets ordinarily nest in or near the ground, although in unusually rainy seasons they may nest higher up, on a porch, for example. If you see them in your neighborhood, try to spot their nesting place. Disturbing a nest can cause the yellow jackets to attack in a swarm. Such accidents are common during gardening, mowing lawns or fields, and while horseback riding through fields.

Brown and black wasps, often found around and in houses, are less inclined to sting. Accidents will happen, however, especially in the spring or fall, if the creatures are a little drowsy from the cold. It is then easy to step on one. They are also apt to lie concealed in clothing or in shoes. Shake out clothing and shoes before putting them on. Finally, keep in mind that wasps are also likely to sting if disturbed when you are painting a house, putting in storm windows, cleaning gutters, and so on. As often as not, it is your hands or head that get the sting. To avoid this, scout the region where you will be working the day before and destroy the nests at night. (Follow the directions on the pesticide carefully.)

Fire-ant bites can usually be identified because the ant grabs onto the skin with its jaws and then, nastily, pivots in a circle, stinging as it goes. In about 24 hours, characteristic little blisters appear at the site.

Fire ants live in Texas, Louisiana, Arkansas, Mississippi, Alabama, Georgia, the Carolinas, and Florida. Up to 60 percent of the human population in these areas is stung yearly, with a 1 percent anaphylaxis rate!

Immunization

People sensitive to insect stings can be immunized, and this usually affords good protection. The immunization procedure for wasps and bees is now more effective than formerly. In the past doctors used whole-body extracts, which did not so reliably build the desired venom immunity, but now the venom itself is used.

The use of venom for immunization was first developed in the 1940s by Mary Hewitt Loveless, one of the leading postwar immunologists. But the method was considered dangerous, and the U.S. Food and Drug Administration did not approve venom immunization until 1979.

Fire-ant allergy still is treated with whole-body extract, but the treatment is nevertheless said to be effective.

An antidote to harvester-ant venom is being developed, using a substance from horned lizards that renders them immune to harvester-ant stings. (In fact, they love to eat the ants.) Reportedly, a few patients have been successfully treated with extract of the saliva of the kissing bug after developing an allergy to this creature.

If you can identify your attacker definitely as a honeybee, yellow jacket, or hornet (or if you have brought the bug in for identification), you can be tested and immunized appropriately. But since there is such a crossover in sensitivity among vespids (yellow jackets, hornets, wasps), your doctor may recommend a mixed-venom extract for that sort of immunization. Also, some doctors will advise tests for all species of apids and vespids, in addition to the insect responsible.

A seemingly obvious allergic sensitivity, based on a severe reaction following a sting, should still be confirmed by skin tests or RAST. Sometimes an apparent anaphylactic reaction is really a severe toxic reaction. In such a case, you should carry epinephrine but need not be immunized.

A strong but strictly local reaction, such as a finger that is very swollen and sore after a sting, is not an indication of susceptibility to anaphylaxis from future stings.

The consensus now is that adults who develop hives in reaction to an insect sting should count that as an anaphylactic reaction and consider getting immunized. However, children who develop hives, but no other anaphylactic symptoms, after a sting, are not considered to need immunization. But this issue is still under study.

Venom immunotherapy shots are administered in basically the same manner as allergy shots. Gradually increasing doses of venom are injected once or twice a week until a maintenance dose is reached. Thereafter the injections are given every four to six weeks.

There is disagreement in the medical community as to whether the shots should be continued indefinitely (i.e., for life) or whether they can be stopped after about five years or after skin tests or RAST show no further sensitivity. More studies are needed to settle the question. Probably someone who is at a special risk of death from anaphylaxis—for example, someone with heart disease—should keep up the shots indefinitely.

What is presently certain is that if you have a history of insect anaphylaxis, you should always be prepared to cope with an emergency reaction. You should carry Adrenalin and you should not hike, canoe, or mountain-climb alone.

Avoidance

Beekeeping is one of the most profitable, easily managed forms of farming for the small entrepreneur, but it is not the career of choice for the insect-allergic person. Unfortunately, beekeepers are likely to become allergic sooner or later because of relatively frequent stings. Important research on bee allergy has been done using the blood of beekeepers.

In addition to not working with bees, allergic persons should be sure there are no bee or wasp nests in or near their homes. It is always best if a nonallergic person gets rid of the nests, but with the products on the market now (powerful, long-distance spray insecticides), the process is pretty safe. Just be sure to follow directions and wait until well after dark before spraying the nests.

Try to get rid of nests as early in spring as possible. The residual pesticide tends to discourage further building, reducing the amount of spray needed later.

Because it can be very difficult to spot ground bees (yellow jackets), be careful about going barefoot, gardening, hiking, mowing, field and trail riding on horses, and other outdoor activities.

If you have wasps flying around your house or just outside, try to locate the nest and get rid of it, rather than just spraying the individuals.

Do not go out in summer wearing scented cosmetics or hygienic products. Do not picnic or snack outdoors. Bees and wasps love soda, sweet iced tea or tea with orange, corn on the cob, watermelon, and other sweet foods.

Do not drink out of doors from soda cans or dark bottles. A bee or wasp may have flown into the container.

Be careful when you are around compost heaps and while handling garbage.

If you have an article of clothing that seems to attract bees (and any strong or bright color or pattern—even black—may do so), do not wear it in daylight during the summer. Neutral shades, such as tan, are safer.

It is best not to have honeysuckle or other very sweet plants near your home.

Be careful when painting a house, cleaning gutters, and so on.

Inspect your car for bees before driving. If a bee flies in while you are on the road, pull over, get out, open the windows and let the creature fly out.

Treatment of Anaphylaxis

For almost all varieties of anaphylaxis, there are basically just two treatments: avoidance and emergency measures. The main exception is insect stings, for which immunization therapy can be used, as we just described above. Very, very occasionally, an effort is made to desensitize a drug-allergic person so that the drug can be used in treatment. This must be done under constant medical supervision in a hospital.

The key in emergency treatment is injection of epinephrine (Adrenalin) as soon as possible after the reaction begins. This acts to stop the release of the chemical mediators of the allergic reaction, and it buys time to get to the hospital or to call medical personnel to the scene. The patient should be in an emergency room or under the care of trained emergency medical technicians within five to 15 minutes of the onset of the attack if possible. A tourniquet can be used to stop the flow of insect venom. Remember, the tourniquet must be loosened for one minute every three minutes.

Epinephrine (Adrenalin) injections can be repeated every 15 minutes. Antihistamines may be added. Intravenous medications and fluid replacement are often indicated. Oxygen therapy and the insertion of a tube into the trachea to keep it open are frequently necessary. Corticosteroids are used to prevent a second-phase reaction later.

Anyone who has had an anaphylactic attack, indeed perhaps anyone in an isolated household, should have at hand emergency epinephrine (Adrenalin) in injectable form. This applies even to patients on venom immunotherapy. We usually speak of having an EpiPen, because that is the device most patients use most easily. There is also an EpiPen Jr. for children. However, some doctors may recommend the Ana-Kit, which contains a syringe and needle and two doses of epinephrine.

You must follow the instructions given with the kit and given by your doctor. In particular, be sure to replace the drug when it expires or as stipulated in the instructions.

You can also keep antihistamines on hand, but these are not very helpful in a life-threatening crisis. It is more important to use epinephrine and to get to an emergency room quickly.

You should also wear a Medic Alert bracelet or carry a card stating that you are allergic and that you have had anaphylaxis, as well as stating the cause of the anaphylaxis.

14

Occupational Allergies and "Sick Buildings"

In the 17th century, Bernardino Ramazzini published a treatise on diseases and disorders that tend to affect workers in various occupations (potters, metal workers, and glaziers, among others). He made the point that breathing noxious fumes and dust appeared to be the cause of many of the ailments associated with these occupations.

Ramazzini's study, *De Morbis Artificum Diatriba,* earned him the title of "father of occupational medicine." This branch of medicine, however, extends back much further than the 18th century. Both Socrates and Hippocrates pointed out the relationship between environment and disease. Also, certain occupations have always been recognized as dangerous and unhealthy.

The most notorious, perhaps, is mining, which was an important occupation even in Neolithic times. Among the ancient Egyptians, mining was a major industry. But only the least fortunate, typically prisoners or prisoners of war and their families, worked in the mines. Their life expectancy was very short.

In literature, a famous example of occupational disease is the affliction of the Mad Hatter in *Alice in Wonderland.* Hatters in the 19th and early 20th centuries were likely to develop neurological disorders as a result of contact with mercury, used in the felting process.

Another heavy metal long recognized as a workplace poison is lead. In 18th-century France, jobs in paint factories, where lead exposure was the norm, were frequently held by ex-convicts, barred by law from many desirable places of residence and types of work. Even today, the lead in paint continues to poison millions of U.S. citizens, primarily children in substandard housing.

Other 20th-century occupational hazards include asbestosis, a crippling, often fatal lung disease, formerly common among those manufacturing and installing asbestos products; pesticide poisoning among migrant farm workers; increased cancer rates among X-ray technicians; and so on.

Allergic or other immune-system reactions to substances in the workplace are ordinarily less serious than the hazards just described, but they frequently indicate a potentially critical health problem in the working environment, such as a contaminated air-conditioning system. Sometimes even allergic reactions, if not recognized and treated, can cause life-threatening damage, usually to the lungs.

Fresh Air

Ramazzini recognized that poor air exchange in the workplace or home made it a great deal more likely that people would sicken. Benjamin Franklin wrote, "No common air from without is so unwholesome as the air within a closed room that has been often breathed and not changed."

Sleeping with the window open, even in the dead of winter, was a health imperative in many English and Yankee households in the 19th century and still is into our own time. Many Continental Europeans, however, held to the view that it is unhealthy to breathe the night air.

There is something to be said for both theories. As we shall see, good air exchange is essential to avoiding pollution of interior air. On the other hand, in many parts of the world, exposure to the night air was and sometimes still is dangerous because of the number of disease-carrying mosquitos active after dark.

Since the 1950s, the trend in architecture has been toward sealed buildings in which natural air flow is replaced by climate-control systems. These systems tend not to function well because of poor design, poor maintenance, poor operation, or all three. The number of allergens, toxins, bacteria, and viruses floating around in the air in some buildings is truly amazing.

In a 1988 article on building-related illnesses in *Clinical Reviews in Allergy* by E. J. Bardana, Jr., Anthony Montanaro, and M.T. O'Hollaren, the authors note that indoor air pollution in the United States became even worse after the energy crisis (oil shortage) of the 1970s. Professional engineering standards for indoor ventilation were reduced from 10 cubic feet replaced per minute per person to 5 cubic feet per minute. Moreover, the 10-cubic-foot standard was itself a reduction from 30 cubic feet per minute, the standard earlier in the century. The American Society of Heating, Refrigerating, and Air-Conditioning Engineers now recommends replacing 20 cubic feet of air per minute per person.

The authors cite an investigation in the 1980s of the General Services Administration Building in Washington, D.C., in which more than 83,000 mold spores per cubic meter were detected. They were coming from slime in the air-conditioner drain pans. "This is comparable to the level of contamination that might be found in a chicken coop," the authors observe.

Among the infectious diseases transmitted through ventilation, heating, and cooling systems is Legionnaires' disease, which killed 29 people staying at the same hotel in Philadelphia in 1976 during an American Legion convention. A similar disease is Pontiac fever. Q fever, usually contracted from animals, also can be transmitted in a building's climate-control system.

Two of the most serious allergic or immunologic diseases caused by substances circulating in closed environments are occupational asthma and hypersensitivity pneumonitis.

Occupational Asthma

Occupational asthma is fairly common, but only a minority of cases are allergic in nature. Nonallergic occupational asthma typically involves the release of chemical mediators that provoke an allergylike response. But the allergy antibody, IgE, does not play a role.

The distinction may seem academic from the patient's point

of view, but making the correct diagnosis of the type of asthma can be important in designing the treatment. Avoidance is usually the treatment of choice, but if the asthma has an allergy component, immunization may be helpful.

The mechanism of nonallergic occupational asthma is not completely known. The harmful substance may irritate nerves in the lungs. Or it may act by opening up the space between cells in the lungs' lining, exposing and stimulating underlying mast cells and the release of chemical mediators. Either way, the result is asthmatic bronchoconstriction and inflammation.

Workers who already have one of the other atopic allergic diseases (allergic rhinitis or atopic dermatitis) are at a greater than normal risk of contracting allergic occupational asthma. This is also true of people with a family history of atopic diseases.

If the asthma is allergic, then the diagnosis can be made by skin tests or RAST. If not, one must narrow the field through a careful case history and other means. Naturally a pattern of illness associated with the workplace is an indicator of the likely diagnosis. The patient may complain of coughing or wheezing at work, sometimes with rhinitis symptoms (sneezing, stuffy nose, burning eyes), then report that at night or on the weekends the symptoms fade. The association is not always so clear, however, because late-phase reactions sometimes take place away from work.

A doctor should ask whether your work exposes you to any of the well-known culprits in occupational asthma. The offending substances that cause allergic asthma very often come from animals. For example, one-fifth of laboratory workers who handle animals have symptoms of allergic rhinitis or allergic asthma related to their work.

Plant proteins also can cause allergic asthma. For example, proteolytic enzymes used in the manufacture of detergents cause adverse reactions in many workers. (Exposure to detergents at home as well as work makes the onset of asthma more likely.) Mold spores from grains, grasses, and wood can also cause asthma.

Rhinitis usually precedes the asthma, so if you are getting symptoms resembling hay fever or a cold at work, try to determine as early as possible whether the problem is exposure to an allergen. You do not want to progress from rhinitis to asthma, so pay attention if your eyes are burning and you are sneezing and sniffling. If the symptoms continue for more than two weeks, see a doctor.

If the problem is exposure to allergens circulated through a humidifier or other climate-control mechanism at work, the diagnosis and treatment can be quite difficult, as they may require the cooperation of management. You may have to change jobs. Ideally, air sampling of the workplace should be done. For many allergens and toxins, the National Institute of Occupational Safety and Health has established guidelines for permissible levels in the air.

Hypersensitivity Pneumonitis

In its acute form, this disease is an explosive reaction to inhaling some type of organic dust or vapor. The disease is just as likely to hit someone who is not allergic as someone who is. Even if you have no allergies and come from an allergy-free family, you may still be affected.

Among the hundreds of inhalants that may cause pneumonitis are numerous plant and animal proteins (as in urine, feces, and dander) as well as mold spores and microorganisms from food, hair, hay, sawdust, and so on.

Pneumonitis is the result of an intense sensitization that can take months or years to develop. But once you have become hypersensitized to a particular substance, you are liable to experience a severe immunologic inflammatory reaction in the lungs if you inhale that substance. This reaction typically occurs within four to six hours after exposure. The symptoms are cough, difficulty breathing, fever (sometimes as high as 104°), with chills and aches. The symptoms may persist up to 18 hours. If the cause of the disease is a sensitivity to bird droppings, there may be a two-phase reaction, with asthmalike symptoms preceding the more typical flulike reaction.

Thermoactinomyces bacteria, found in damp hay, straw, and other vegetation, can also infest certain air-conditioning and humidifying systems (including room humidifiers in which stagnant water and debris collect). When this substance vaporizes and is circulated, it can cause hypersensitivity pneumonitis, called in this case ventilation pneumonitis.

Recovery from a pneumonitis attack is spontaneous, but the

symptoms will reappear at the next exposure. Repeated attacks may lead to loss of appetite, weight loss, and severe breathlessness.

Diagnosis

A doctor listening to your chest during an acute attack will probably hear distinctive sounds called rales. Blood studies are likely to show an increase in immunoglobulins and white blood cells, as if you had a severe infection. Pulmonary function may be markedly changed from your normal performance.

Unpleasant as all this may be, at least the severity of the symptoms tends to drive people to seek medical help. Unfortunately, there is a chronic form of hypersensitivity pneumonitis, in which the patient suffers similar but very mild symptoms. Often the main sign of trouble is nothing more than a nagging cough, which seems like some kind of stubborn bronchitis. The signs of chronic pneumonitis are shortness of breath and weight loss over time. In the meanwhile the lungs are becoming fibrotic (scarred). They can become so damaged, in fact, that the patient may die.

Obviously it is important not to ignore persistent health problems. There is always a reason for a cough and breathlessness. It may be minor or it may be critical, but it should be found.

In order to establish the diagnosis, it may be necessary to run special challenge tests using the suspect substance, such as debris from a humidifier, or, if the patient is a farmer, dust from moldy hay. Such tests are usually done in a hospital. After inhaling the suspect substance the patient is monitored for 24 hours on a variety of factors, including pulmonary function. A lung biopsy may be helpful in checking for lung-tissue damage.

Treatment

Treatment of hypersensitivity pneumonitis is first of all avoidance of the offending substance. Sometimes improved ventilation, air filtration, a cleaning of the climate-control system, or wearing a breathing mask can provide adequate protection. But a change of occupation, job, or residence may be necessary.

Pharmaceutical treatment centers on the administration of

oral corticosteroids (cortisone), but steroid treatment should never be substituted for avoidance, since it does not halt the progress of the disease when there is chronic exposure.

Workers at Risk

The following are some of the occupations in which one may be exposed to substances causing hypersensitivity pneumonitis.

Animal Workers

People who work with animals in laboratories, veterinary offices, farms, or elsewhere, or who simply have pets, may develop allergic asthma or hypersensitivity pneumonitis from exposure to the dander, urine, or feces of the animals. People working with birds, for instance, may develop what is called pigeon breeder's (or bird breeder's) disease, or hen worker's disease. The dried feces of pigeons, parakeets, chickens, and other birds can enter the air and be inhaled, causing hypersensitivity pneumonitis. Similarly, jockeys are more likely than those in the general population to come down with asthma.

Bakers

Baker's asthma, which affects as many as 10 percent of bakers, may be caused by allergenic proteins in flour and grains. Fungi of the *Aspergillus* and *Alternaria* genuses and other organisms have also been linked to baker's asthma. The disease, which may take years to develop, is usually preceded by allergic rhinitis, and there seems to be a genetic aspect—that is, those from atopic families are more likely to get it.

Cosmeticians and Hairdressers

The beauty business is not all glamour. Hairdressers have been reported to develop rhinitis and asthma as a result of allergy to human hair or dander. Persulfates in bleach can cause asthma, and many other chemicals used in treating hair and in cosmetics cause both respiratory and skin reactions.

Detergent Workers

A sensitivity to subtilisin (an animal enzyme in detergents) can cause respiratory distress among people involved in manufacturing detergents. Exposure at home can also be an inciting factor in the development or continuation of the illness.

Dockworkers and Granary Workers

Grains of all sorts contain allergens that may affect the sensitive person, leading to asthma and eventually, if untreated, to serious lung disease. "Grain fever" is essentially the same as baker's asthma.

Farmers

Farmers are frequently exposed to bacteria in wet baled hay. When inhaled, the bacteria can produce hypersensitivity pneumonitis, sometimes called farmer's lung. Straw and grains may contain the same bacteria (of the *Thermoactinomyces* species). The disease often occurs in the winter, when the farmer works with old hay in a closed barn.

Farmers who handle animals are susceptible to the afflictions of animal workers described above.

Food Processors and Cooks

People preparing many kinds of food develop allergic rhinitis and asthma.

Allergies to plant proteins and plant enzymes also afflict food processors. Mushroom worker's disease is a type of hypersensitivity pneumonitis, and is secondary to exposure to *Thermoactinomyces* bacteria.

Dust from coffee beans and cocoa beans can also be a fairly potent allergen, as can moldy malt, in which the allergen *Aspergillus* mold may be present. The result is malt worker's disease.

Cheese worker's lung is caused by an allergy to cheese mold. Sensitivity to eggs can cause allergy symptoms among food processors, bakers, and cooks. Simply inhaling vapors of a food to which one is allergic can set off a reaction.

Meat packers occasionally develop asthma from inhaling the

vapors of the polyvinyl plastic wrap used to package meat in supermarkets. The fumes, which come from heating the plastic to seal the wrap, can be avoided by using a wrap that can be sealed without heating.

Furriers and Taxidermists

People working with fur and pelts are prone to a number of infections and adverse reactions caused by the pathogens in fur or by chemicals used to prepare the furs. These problems are difficult to avoid, even when strict cleanliness is practiced.

Metalworkers and Welders

Sensitivity to fumes from heated galvanized steel may cause "metal fume fever" among welders. The symptoms are respiratory distress and fever. Allergic asthma is an occupational hazard among those involved with processing and plating chromium, nickel, or platinum.

Paint and Ink Manufacturers and Painters

Asthma caused by castor-bean dust is a hazard in the manufacture of substances such as certain paints, varnishes, inks, and cosmetics, which use the castor bean. Painters and woodworkers also may develop lung disease due to sensitivity to these substances.

Pharmaceutical Workers

The same allergic sensitivity that causes some people to have adverse reactions to penicillin and other antibiotics affects workers in the pharmaceutical industry who inhale dust or vapors from these drugs.

Plastics, Glue, and Chemical Workers

Diisocynates (such as toluene-2,4-diisocynate, or TDI) used in the manufacture of various chemicals, foam, plastics, and adhesives can cause allergic asthma and, less commonly, hypersensitivity pneumonitis. Workers exposed to these chemicals include not only those in factories, but also spray-painters, people who work with plastic food wrappings, and many others. Reactions to epoxy resins afflict both plastics workers and woodworkers. Exposure to fish-based glue, which is common among bookbinders and postal workers, can cause reactions in people allergic to fish.

Potters and Other Artists

Potter's lung, a reaction to clay dust, is only one of many dozens of ailments that affect artists. Clay, glazes, paints, solvents, fixatives, metal fumes, inks, and so on all are likely to produce adverse toxic or immunological reactions, some permanent or fatal. When buying art materials for children, be sure that they are nontoxic.

Two organizations that provide information on safety in art materials are:

Center for Safety in the Arts, 5 Beekman Street, Suite 1030, New York, NY 10038. Telephone (212) 227-6220.
Arts, Crafts, and Theater Safety, 181 Thompson Street, No. 23, New York, NY 10012. Questions answered by telephone, (212) 777-0062.

Printers

Printing involves exposure to a variety of chemical fumes and vegetable gums that may cause allergic respiratory or skin disorders.

Refrigeration and Air-conditioning Workers

Exposure to microorganisms, especially the bacteria *Micropolyspora* and *Thermoactinomyces,* can lead to humidifier lung, or air-conditioner lung. These are essentially manifestations of humidifier fever. (See "Sick-Building Syndrome," below.)

Sugar-cane Workers

Bagasse is, collectively, fibers and residue remaining after sugar canes are crushed for syrup. Sensitivity to *Micropolyspora* and *Thermoactinomyces* in the bagasse causes sugar-cane worker's fever, or bagassosis. This can lead to hypersensitivity pneumonitis. Sugar-cane workers, especially the cutters, are among the most oppressed of all laborers in the Western Hemisphere, and this is only one of many serious ills to which they are prey; others include pneumonia, tuberculosis, and gangrene.

Textile-mill Workers

Byssinosis, sometimes called mill fever, is a lung disease common among workers exposed to cotton fibers, flax, or hemp. The symptoms are breathlessness, wheezing, cough, and often fever. If not treated for the disease, even an initially healthy person may eventually become very ill with respiratory blockage and emphysema. The condition can be fatal.

It is believed that the cause may be at least in part a sensitivity to toxins produced by bacteria in the plant fibers.

Woodworkers and Builders

Sawmill workers, carpenters, and furniture makers are exposed to wood dust and to a variety of strong chemicals used to treat and finish wood. The dust of Western red cedar, probably the most-studied wood dust, is a well-documented cause of asthma. The substance in the wood causing the harm is believed to be plicatic acid. Unfortunately, years may pass before the asthma recedes, even after no further exposure to the dust. Wood molds can also cause respiratory damage. Sequoiasis, a type of pneumonitis, is caused by moldy redwood.

Sick-building Syndrome

There are some modern buildings where the tight, energy-efficient, but low-ventilation system results in polluted, contaminated air. In such buildings infectious organisms in the climate-control systems and even in water pipes and shower heads can cause serious respiratory disease.

Asthma, hypersensitivity pneumonitis, and allergic bronchopulmonary aspergillosis (see p. 122) may also be caused by exposure to allergens and toxins in the workplace.

Skin symptoms, such as a rash, itching, and sore, burning eyes (especially among those who wear contact lenses), can be the result of fiberglass or wool particles in the air. The former may come from the lining of ventilation ducts.

In addition, the so-called sick-building syndrome usually involves complaints by many workers of headache, fatigue, and irritation of the upper respiratory tract, with cough, sore throat, burning eyes, stuffy or runny nose, and chest tightness. In a humid, inadequately ventilated space, dust mites tend to thrive, causing an increased incidence of allergic rhinitis and asthma. Some workers may suffer toxic or allergic reactions to chemicals not cleared from the air, including cigarette smoke, and fumes and carbon monoxide from an oil-burning furnace. Mold circulating in the air can cause allergies. A high level of carbon dioxide from exhaled air can be a sign that the building is inadequately ventilated. Pesticides used by exterminators can cause toxic reactions and illness. Carpet cleaners can leave behind an irritating chemical residue.

Because of the variety of responses to airborne contaminants, it can be difficult to determine whether the underlying cause of an outbreak of illnesses is related to the design of the workplace or has some other cause. In some instances OSHA (the Occupational Safety and Health Administration) or a state-level counterpart will conduct tests to ascertain conditions within the building. Insurance companies, especially the company that writes disability insurance for the firm, often have a staff of engineers and industrial hygienists who investigate buildings insured by their company.

Humidifier Fever

Humidifier fever is sometimes categorized as a type of hypersensitivity pneumonitis, approximately identical to "ventilation fever." But the term can also be used generally to refer to flulike reactions to molds, bacteria, and other contaminants spread by humidifying systems. The disease may have an asthma component. Typically, when a workplace humidifier is involved, the symptoms—which can include fever, chills, headaches, chest tightness, and shortness of breath—flare up early in the week and subside when one has time off.

Formaldehyde and Other Construction Materials

Use of formaldehyde has declined in recent years, since it has been shown to have a carcinogenic effect. No longer are high school biology labs filled with that unforgettable odor from barrels of formaldehyde and dead frogs awaiting dissection. Nevertheless, formaldehyde is still used in no-press textiles, plywood, and a number of other construction and furnishing materials, including materials for drapes and carpets. It is believed to be the cause of numerous adverse reactions (evidently not IgE-mediated), including bronchitis, hives and rashes, and headaches.

There is a certain amount of skepticism in the medical community concerning reports of formaldehyde sensitivity. Nevertheless, chemicals entering the air from construction materials or textiles must be on the list of suspects when one encounters the sick-building syndrome.

In an embarrassing incident in 1988, workers at the Environmental Protection Agency building in Washington, D.C., fell ill with flulike symptoms, sore throats, and burning lips. Apparently, the new carpet being installed was poisoning the workers. The chemical most likely to have caused the problem was identified as 4-PCH, a by-product of the latex used in carpet backing and glue. This chemical is now being used less in carpet backings, and manufacturers are said to be airing out their products more thoroughly before installation. Nevertheless, during carpet installation it is advisable to keep a good flow of air through the area being carpeted.

It is not possible to avoid all the hazards that might arise from exposure to chemicals in construction materials and office furnishings. But if you or your coworkers have a problem with a particular product, the U.S. Consumer Product Safety Commission may be able to provide relevant information. Their number is (800) 638-2772.

15

Psychological Aspects of Allergy

With any chronic disease, especially when the symptoms are relatively mild, the person affected is probably going to have to put up with an occasional suspicion on the part of family or friends that the ailment is "psychological." This is true of lower back pain (which always seems to flare up at the worst moments), mild arthritis, ulcers, and of course allergies.

Actually, there very likely is a psychological component to all or most diseases. If you have suffered a loss or shock, such as death of a spouse or unexpected unemployment, you are at greater risk of developing any number of diseases, including cancer.

There also seems to be a conditioning mechanism at work in some types of allergy. With hay fever, for example, research has shown that if you have been exposed to a potent allergen in a particular locale, you may undergo an allergic reaction upon returning to that place, even if the allergen is no longer present. This is a conditioned response.

In an experiment with asthmatics allergic to cats, a significant number showed changes in pulmonary function when inhaling a solution in a nebulizer that they were told contained cat dander but that did not.

In perhaps the most surprising experimental result in this field, laboratory rats were given intradermal skin tests for various allergens and then certain musical sounds were played for 48 hours as the tests developed. Subsequently, animals who tested positive were subjected to the same test—but using only a water solution—and the same musical sounds. The animals tested positive to the water.

The interaction between the mind and the immune system is stronger than generally realized. But this does not mean that the immune system's reaction in a conditioned response is "psychological" rather than physical. In these conditioned allergic responses, your sensory and neural systems convey the message "allergen danger," and your immune system responds with protective mechanisms, such as mucus production, bronchial constriction, mast-cell activation in the skin, and so on.

This is not a neurotic response. It is as normal a physical reaction as any other. It does not mean that the disease is "just in your head" or that you can cure it if you "really want to." It means that our thoughts and emotions and the functioning of our bodies are inextricably intertwined.

The role of the psyche in disease is one of the world's most debated questions. Luckily, one need not resolve it in order to use medical information constructively. For example, the symptoms of an asthma attack and the symptoms of an anxiety reaction are very similar. All too many people get in serious trouble with asthma because they try to "just calm down" when they should be calling a taxi or ambulance and heading for the hospital. If you have asthma, don't analyze the cause of the attack; treat the symptoms.

Asthma Mimic

Curiously, there is in fact a disorder that mimics an asthma attack and is due primarily to anxiety. This relatively rare disorder involves a panic dysfunction of the vocal cords, in which the cords move in the wrong direction on exhalation, temporarily blocking air. The patient, who appears to be in danger of choking to death, would benefit at that moment from professional reassurance and distraction designed to give the vocal cords an opportunity to relax and assume a normal position. Instead, patients are often subject to extreme emergency treatment, including intubation (for a respirator) or tracheotomy.

There are several ways of differentiating between vocal-cord (glottal) dysfunction and an asthma attack. With vocal-cord dysfunction, patients can speak and hold their breath. If asked to cough, the patient can do so, and this response may actually set the vocal cords right, relieving the attack. In asthma attacks, patients cannot speak well and get worse if asked to hold their breath or cough. Another diagnostic test is that people with glottal dysfunction are not adversely affected by breathing mecholyl in a challenge test, whereas asthmatics begin to wheeze.

The most effective treatment for glottal dysfunction is psychological counseling to help the patient overcome the anxiety or tension that causes the vocal cords to malfunction. Breathing training and voice training may also help. Most asthmatics, however, will not benefit from this approach, although learning breathing and relaxation techniques may be generally useful in helping the patient cope with the disease.

The allergy diseases that seem to be influenced most frequently by one's psychological state are eczema, hives, and allergic asthma. There is no scientific estimate of what percentage of patients having these diseases might experience an improvement through reducing stress or increasing happiness, but a guess based on years of experience is that about one-third may be in that category. This third would include children. We often forget how stressful children's lives can be. Some children are severely depressed, and a recent study has indicated that depression in asthmatic children significantly increases their risk of dying of the disease.

Stress

The major villain among psychological causes of physical disease is stress. The stress can be physical as well as psychological in origin. For example, a maltreated child who is physically abused is also emotionally stressed. The overworked single parent may be both sleep-deprived and chronically anxious over how to make financial ends meet.

People vary enormously in how much stress they can tolerate. Some are bored without constant pressure and challenges. Some need to work quietly, with lots of time to relax. Most at risk of suffering serious adverse effects from stress are those who physiologically do not handle stress very well—their blood pressure rises, for example—even though they may not consciously sense this reaction at all. They appear calm and they feel calm, but they are heading for a medical crisis.

Pioneer studies of the physical effects of stress were carried out in the 1930s by Hans Selye. He reported that rats who were severely stressed showed changes in their adrenal glands and in their immune systems, and developed gastrointestinal ulcers.

The initial changes that take place in reaction to stress (a surge of adrenaline, increased heart rate, and so on) are designed to help you to overcome or escape a dangerous or painful situation, whether it be social (such as a sadistic boss at work) or physical (a bad automobile accident). But if the pain cannot be overcome or avoided, and the stress is severe, most people will eventually suffer exhaustion and dysfunction in one or more body systems.

Fear and anger act on the autonomic nervous system, which controls the functioning of internal organs and blood and lymph vessels, but it is not known why some people under stress are affected in one organ system rather than another—why, for example, some develop stomach ulcers while others develop respiratory illnesses. Possibly an original imbalance in the biochemistry of an organ makes it prone to dysfunction under stress.

With respect to asthma, stress lowers the level of the neurotransmitter CAMP, a substance that asthmatics need, for it counteracts bronchoconstriction and the release of histamine and other chemical mediators by the mast cells. Through its effect on the mast cells, the reduction in CAMP may also play a role in outbreaks of eczema, hives, and rhinitis (see chapter 12).

There is a type of perennial rhinitis, vasomotor rhinitis, that is similar to perennial allergic rhinitis, except that no allergic factor can be found. Psychological factors may play a role in this disorder.

Stress also seems to play a role in the causation of chronic hives, although it is not the only cause. There is less evidence that stress influences acute hives.

Medicines and Mood Changes

Being sick undermines one's psychological well-being. People who have never suffered an asthma attack have difficulty appreciating how frightening and at the same time infuriating these episodes can be. No one is at their best when trying to cope with repeated episodes of what may be a life-threatening illness. To add to the patient's psychological burden, the medicines prescribed may cause mood changes as well.

Antihistamines, of course, are widely used in the treatment of allergies and are famous for producing lethargy. Paradoxically, in some patients, especially children, antihistamines may stimulate the central nervous system, causing anxiety, difficulty sleeping, and restlessness. The H2 antihistamines, especially cimetidine (Tagamet), have been associated with confusion in elderly patients. Alcohol and other recreational drugs are likely to exaggerate these side effects.

As noted in the chapter on therapeutic drugs, many of the problems traditionally associated with antihistamines can be avoided by using the new, nonsoporific preparations, such as terfenadine (Seldane) and astemizole (Hismanal).

Several of the drugs used to treat asthma and occasionally other severe allergic conditions may cause restlessness, anxiety, shakiness, and difficulty concentrating. The most tricky to handle are the corticosteroids, which may have to be taken over long periods. They can cause mood swings from agitation to depression and may even, although rarely, produce psychotic symptoms. Withdrawal can lead to depression, and for both physical and psychological reasons it should always be gradual.

Theophylline, which is often prescribed for both children and adults with asthma, is related to caffeine. The effects are variable, but jumpiness and difficulty concentrating are common. Needless to say, this may affect a child's schoolwork.

Beta 2 agonists and epinephrine may cause tremors and anxiety. Ephedrine, too, is a stimulant and may increase alertness, but it also may cause insomnia and irritability.

Some allergy patients, typically older patients, are also regularly taking medications other than those prescribed for the allergy. Your doctors and your pharmacist should be aware of every medicine you may be taking.

Ask what precautions you should observe, what side effects to watch out for, and what is the best way to take each medication: With food? At night? Write down the information and keep it with your medicines. Do not feel embarrassed to ask these questions again frequently. New information on the effects of drugs is constantly being discovered.

Treatment

In the 12th century, Maimonides wrote of the asthma patient: "In mental anguish, fear, mourning or distress, his agitation affects his respiratory organs, and he cannot exercise them at will. . . . The cure lies not in foods, in drugs alone, nor in regular medical advice; psychological methods are a greater help."

In our time, however, at the height of the enthusiasm for Freudian theory, the insight that emotions influence health was sometimes given too much weight. In the 1950s, for example, all too many people with treatable organic disorders were spending time and money on psychoanalysis that was not helping. Patients who deserved sympathy and effective medical treatment were at risk of being told how neurotic they were. Certain personality types were said to have a tendency to develop certain illnesses.

The medical community is now trying to strike a balance in its approach to treatment. Instead of tending to think that certain personality types are to "blame" for certain illnesses, there is attention to research that suggests that often it is the illness itself that alters the personality, producing the suspect characteristics. Today, rather than assuming that psychological disturbance underlies every allergic illness, the focus is more on the particular patient. Your doctor should consider and discuss with you whether stress or lifestyle may play a role in your allergy flare-ups.

To alleviate the anxiety that naturally comes with being sick, ask your doctor for information about the mood swings that ordinarily accompany illness or use of certain medicines. This holds for a child patient as well as an adult. Both parent and child should have an understanding of how the disease and the treatment may affect their feelings and ability to concentrate and work. If you feel that your moods are becoming difficult to handle or that your personality is changing, as the result either of medication or of the disease itself, you have a right to expect a sympathetic and helpful response from your doctor.

Keep in mind, however, that, in order to provide effective help, the doctor may have to ask about work conditions, family life, drinking or smoking habits, and other issues that ordinarily are private. It may be that an unhappy child should change schools or that an adult should join Alcoholics Anonymous.

If an intractable problem is identified, your doctor should be able to recommend for your consideration family counseling, a smoking clinic, psychiatric therapy, or whatever is indicated.

To protect your interests, you should ask a therapist what results should emerge from the treatment and how long the process will take. If the treatment is goal-oriented, you will be better able to assess whether it is working or not.

You might think that since some allergy responses apparently can be conditioned, therefore behavior-oriented conditioning treatment would be especially promising. But the value of such conditioning has not been established. It is far easier to transfer a response to different situations than to eliminate it.

For example, in the classic conditioning experiment, Pavlov's dogs "learned" to salivate upon hearing a bell, because many times in the past that bell had sounded as food was given. One can retrain such dogs so that they do not salivate when a bell rings, but training them not to salivate at feeding time would be another story.

If most of your allergy symptoms are unconditioned—that is, if they are direct responses to allergens in the environment (just as salivating is a direct response to food)—then behavior or conditioning therapy may not be much help.

Turning to other modes of treatment, there is not much scientific evidence to show that psychoanalysis, the various forms of psychotherapy, or hypnosis has much effect on the progress of asthma or other allergic conditions. Nevertheless, as we have mentioned, for some people the emotional support of a psychotherapist through this stressful illness can be helpful. Therapists who have a good record in curing panic attacks and phobias may be able to provide some help in reducing anxiety reactions associated with allergic asthma and other allergic diseases.

Physical exercise and some of the relaxation and breathing exercises done in yoga and other, similar types of discipline are beneficial to many patients. Of course, if you are under a doctor's care, you should discuss any exercise or sports program with her or him before getting started. Vigorous exercise has both physical and psychological rewards for asthmatics, although it must be carefully managed (see chapter 9). Fresh air, adequate sleep, and a good, healthful diet are also important in coping with almost any illness.

16

Allergies in Children

Allergies in infants and toddlers are almost always handled by the baby's pediatrician, which is appropriate. A good pediatrician is qualified to diagnose and treat most allergies in infants and young children. Allergists are rarely called in for children under age two, unless the case is unusually troublesome—for example, if the child has multiple allergies or allergic asthma.

Later in childhood, however, allergists often take an active role in treatment. One of the main types of allergy treatment, immunotherapy (allergy shots), is more likely to be successful in the 5–25 age group than in any other, and is almost always undertaken by an allergist.

There are a couple of reasons for waiting until a child is about five to do immunotherapy. There is some concern that the immune system of younger children may not be adequately mature for such treatment and that complications, including anaphylaxis, might arise. Also, it is often not possible to be certain at so young an age that the symptoms will persist.

Nevertheless, in some cases in which an allergy is clearly established, immunotherapy, or allergy shots, may be recommended for a child under age five, and may work very well.

Children's Allergies to Food and Drugs

Allergy to cow's milk is so common among young children that it is one of the many reasons to breast-feed. Caring for a baby with milk allergy is no fun. Common symptoms are diarrhea, stomach pain, and rashes. Moreover, in the first few weeks of life, breast milk also provides protection against respiratory, gastrointestinal, and meningeal (meningitis) infections.

Soy formula is the standard substitute for cow's milk, but it is costly and some babies do not like the taste. If the baby develops an allergy to soy as well, a more expensive formula based on meat or other proteins will have to be tried.

One hypoallergenic formula on the market is Nutramigen (Mead Johnson Pharmaceuticals), a highly predigested casein formula. A similar, less predigested but also less expensive hypoallergenic formula is Good Start (Carnation). Some children do well on goat's milk, although this is rarely used today.

If there is a family history of allergies, or if your baby has already shown signs of allergy, discuss with your pediatrician the advisability of delaying or limiting the addition of solid food to the baby's diet.

Can Allergy in Infancy Be Prevented by Altering the Diet of the Mother in Pregnancy?

Allergists have been intrigued by the idea that altering the diet of a mother during pregnancy could alter the development of allergic disease in a child with a potential to develop allergies. There is presently no sound scientific evidence that alteration of the diet during any stage of pregnancy will affect the allergic state of the developing fetus. However, this matter is still under investigation; therefore, if you are pregnant or about to become pregnant, and there are allergies in your family or the father's, be sure to discuss this problem with your allergist and obstetrician. For a more precise definition of which children are at risk of becoming allergic, see below.

Alteration of the Allergic State After Birth

Recently evidence has been put forth that alteration of the child's diet in the first year of life can very significantly delay and reduce the incidence of allergic disease in the allergic child. However, first we must identify what we mean by the allergic child. We agree with Dr. Robert S. Ziegler, an associate professor of pediatrics at the University of California at San Diego and an acknowledged expert on this subject, that the infants who can be helped by dietary adjustments are those with (1) both parents allergic or (2) one parent allergic and at least one other sibling also allergic.

Such a child can benefit from breast-feeding for four to six months. During the time the child is breast-feeding, the mother should consult with a pediatrician on dietary matters. In general, she should avoid allergenic foods (eggs, milk, peanuts) and should supplement her diet with 1,500 mg of elemental calcium to make up for the lack of calcium in the milk that she can't drink.

Soy formula can be just as allergenic as milk. Therefore, if the baby needs a supplement, use a protein hydrolysate formula, such as Nutramigen. Do not introduce any of the allergenic solid foods until after the first year of age. Then the following allergenic foods should be added cautiously, if tolerated, at the rate of one every other week: milk, wheat, soy, corn, citrus, eggs, peanuts, fish. Delay eggs, peanuts, and fish even longer if the child has already shown signs of food allergy.

Foods other than milk are best added to a baby's diet one by one, starting with the least allergenic foods (rice cereal and scraped banana). If a food allergy develops, the problem food should be withdrawn, although in a year or two the child may grow out of the sensitivity. Eggs, fruit, chocolate, wheat, orange juice and other acid fruit, and shellfish are common causes of allergic reactions in infants and young children.

Be cautious about concluding on informal evidence that a child is allergic to sweets, "nonorganic" foods, or any other type of food. If you observe that your child does not do well on certain foods, try to keep them out of the child's diet. But before determining that a food should be eliminated altogether, get medical advice. The effects of overly restricting a child's food choices, particularly if based on unproven theories, can create their own problems.

If healthy food makes up the bulk of the child's diet, and you do not routinely stock sodas, salty snacks, and candy, then a small dessert and a cookie or two each day will do no harm.

Anaphylactic reactions to food are rare in childhood. But if one occurs, the child must be taught never again to eat the food that caused the reaction. Set an example by reading food labels with the child and asking questions in restaurants. If the child eats meals at school, be sure that the nutritionist knows of the youngster's allergy and supervises food preparation and consumption accordingly. Notify the school nurse as well.

A child who has had an anaphylactic reaction should carry an EpiPen and wear or carry a Medic Alert bracelet or similar identification so that people will recognize a medical emergency if it occurs.

Allergies to eggs and milk tend to disappear after age five, but other allergies, such as to peanuts, tree nuts, and shellfish, tend to last a lifetime. After a number of years have passed, an allergist may recommend a challenge test in a hospital or similarly safe setting to determine if the allergy is still present. The chapters on food and drug allergies contain more information on these subjects.

From a psychological perspective, it is important as far as possible not to make an allergic child feel or appear different from other children. Food allergies should be treated matter-of-factly.

You can help teach a child who absolutely must avoid one or more foods the social skills that will help him or her get through difficult times. A young person who talks incessantly about his or her allergies will soon have many social problems. Kids with smooth manners learn to sound regretful about having to pass on an offered food. Other children's parents are often not sympathetic enough to the needs of a small visitor with allergies.

As for over-the-counter medicines, it is best not to use any one medicine frequently without checking with your pediatrician or family doctor. Some should not be used on children at all. Aspirin is a wonderful drug but is rarely recommended now for people under age 18; if given in association with certain viral infections, it may cause Reye's syndrome (a disease affecting the brain and other internal organs). Aspirin sensitivity, associated with asthma and allergy reactions, such as hives, is also common.

If your child is treated with penicillin or another antibiotic, be aware of the possibility that an allergy may develop. In very rare cases an allergy reaction may appear on first exposure. In most or all such cases, there probably has been covert prior exposure in food or by some other means.

If a child is given a shot of any kind, it is best to keep the child in the doctor's office, or at least within reach of medical help, for a half hour in case an anaphylactic reaction occurs. Sometimes a child who is allergic to a drug or serum will complain of a sore throat or will vomit, and the parent mistakenly assumes these symptoms are due to the sickness for which the youngster is being treated or are a normal reaction to the shot.

In the hour or so following your child's injection, pay close attention to any complaints involving a sore or swollen mouth or throat, itching or swelling anywhere on the body, hives, or difficulty speaking. If these symptoms start to appear following a shot, immediately bring the child back to the doctor's office or to an emergency room.

Rashes and Hives

Certain reactions affecting the skin are particularly common among young children.

As just noted, children are prone to food sensitivities, many of which pass as time goes on. A common symptom is an outbreak of hives, and acute hives occur more often among children than adults.

Not surprisingly, diaper dermatitis, or diaper rash, affects the younger set almost exclusively. It results from leaving the baby too long in soiled diapers or from using diapers in which there is a residue of soap or antiseptic. The condition's distinguishing characteristic is that it affects the skin under the diaper and the adjacent areas of the stomach and thighs.

The first step in treatment is to keep the child as clean and dry as possible. Change the diaper frequently and wash the baby with mild soap and water—rinse well. If you are using cloth diapers, give them an extra rinse to be sure that they are clean.

Use only a mild soap. If you are using a diaper service, and you believe that soap or detergent is the problem, notify them.

The rash will clear up more quickly if you use plain cloth diapers, without rubber pants or a plastic outer layer. Better yet, let the baby go without diapers if possible.

Zinc oxide cream helps to protect young skin. A 1 percent hydrocortisone cream is often effective in healing the rash, although use of this or stronger topical steroids should be approved by a doctor. The stronger preparations should not be used for more than a week unless the condition is severe, which is not usually the case with simple diaper rash. If the symptoms persist for several days, the baby should be seen by a doctor. There is always a possibility of bacterial or fungal infection, and other, more serious, skin diseases are occasionally mistaken for diaper dermatitis.

Atopic Dermatitis

Atopic dermatitis (eczema) can flare in infancy and throughout early childhood. In the past, many children endured long, miserable periods of eczema, during which they were swathed in compresses and told not to scratch or were restrained to prevent scratching.

Modern corticosteroids, although they must be used with great care, have taken much of the agony out of severe eczema. It is very important to remember, however, how potent these drugs are. Your doctor should not be casual about supervising treatment, and it is essential to pay close attention to medical directions from your doctor, from the pharmacist, and on the label.

Atopic dermatitis usually does not appear before the child is two months old. In the youngest children it is apt to appear first on the face, especially on the cheeks. Later it may spread to the area of the hairline and behind the ears (see chapter 12).

The disease may clear up in infancy, but sometimes it progresses or reappears after a time of remission. Among toddlers and older children, the rash (dry lesions) characteristically appears in front of the elbows, where the arms bend, and behind the knees. The face is often spared, but the feet may not be, and the rash may be misdiagnosed as athlete's foot. In adoles-

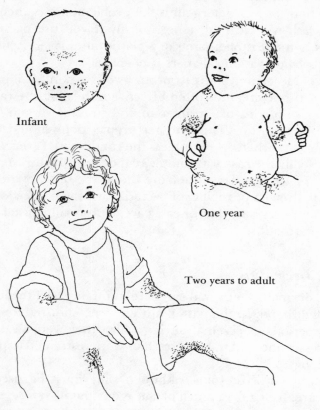

Infant

One year

Two years to adult

Distribution of Atopic Dermatitis in Children

cence the rash often becomes milder. Unfortunately, it occasionally becomes much worse and widespread, affecting large areas of the head, neck, chest, arms, and feet.

Statistically, more than half of children with atopic dermatitis at age three will still have the condition as adults. And as you probably know at this point in the book, the atopic diseases (allergic rhinitis, atopic dermatitis, and asthma) run in families, and if you have one, you may develop another. Up to three-quarters of youngsters with atopic dermatitis develop allergic rhinitis or asthma, but it is rare to have all three.

Children who have developed atopic dermatitis and are therefore at risk of developing asthma may get some protection through control of their exposure to allergens. *Reducing exposure to dust mites, and perhaps mold, dander, and cockroaches as well, may prevent the development of asthma in these children.* Similar precautions may be helpful for all children whose parents are allergic.

The treatment of atopic dermatitis is the same for children as for adults (see chapter 12).

Contact Dermatitis

Children's skin is very delicate. Most of us can remember the awful discomfort of itchy woolen sweaters or trousers. If a child says that a piece of clothing makes him or her itch, believe it.

Wool is an irritant in and of itself, but chemicals used in the processing of fabrics and the manufacture of clothing can also cause contact dermatitis, especially in places where the garment fits tightly. Sometimes washing or cleaning new clothes before wearing them solves the problem.

Poison-ivy resin can imbue a fabric or be carried on an animal's coat for several days, with the potential of causing poison-ivy dermatitis if the resin touches the skin. Teach your children to recognize and avoid this plant and to put clothing in the wash if they have been walking through poison ivy. If a pet has been running through poison ivy, the animal should not be hugged and kissed until it has had a bath.

Other plants, including chrysanthemums, can cause contact dermatitis. The disease also can be caused by substances containing plant products, such as turpentine and Vicks VapoRub.

Some children react to leather or rubber used in shoes or to nickel in the toes of certain shoes by developing contact dermatitis. To make diagnosis more difficult, atopic dermatitis caused by something as remote as a food allergy may also cause a rash on the feet.

At any rate, if it is contact dermatitis patch tests can identify the offending substance. Sometimes protective socks (such as those made from thick cotton) solve the problem. Occasionally, one must order special shoes not containing the allergen.

Children can be sensitive to over-the-counter medications used to treat cuts, insect bites, sunburn, and the like. The preparations most frequently causing reactions are those with "-caine" in the ingredients (for example, benzocaine), topical antihistamines and antibiotics, and ethylenediamine (used as a solvent and emulsifier in a number of medical compounds).

Contact dermatitis around the mouth, often confused with atopic dermatitis, is commonly caused by licking the lips. Acid foods, such as oranges and juices, can dry around the mouth and irritate the skin. Rubber erasers can cause contact dermatitis around the lips.

Allergic Rhinitis–Related Conditions in Children

Allergic rhinitis is an all-too-common childhood disease. When combined with the usual quota of head colds in childhood, this one-two punch can leave kids with runny noses for a good portion of their young lives.

Children with allergic rhinitis tend to develop an "allergic look." They often have buck teeth from propping open their mouths with a thumb or fingers to breathe in more air. Their eyes may be dark-circled, with so-called allergic shiners. Frequently there is a crease between the tip and bridge of the nose as a result of pushing up the snub of the nose in the "allergic salute," which is a vigorous wiping of the nose.

Serial sneezing, an itching palate, allergic conjunctivitis, and coughing round out the most common symptoms.

Needless to say, the popularity of children with allergic rhinitis can be affected by these miserable symptoms. Some children who live with untreated allergies do well in school and sports, and are well liked. But most need medical attention to be and do their best.

An important first step in most cases is to make the child's room allergen-free (see chapter 4). This sometimes leads to a dramatic improvement, whether the offending culprit is an indoor allergen such as dust mites or whether it is pollen or mold from outside. A recent article in the *New England Journal of Medicine* suggests that it might be a good idea to provide a mite-free environment for children in high-risk families (families in which one or both parents have a history of allergic diseases—allergic rhinitis, asthma, or eczema). Ridding the house of dust mites is a good idea; the same may apply to mold spores, dander, and cockroaches.

If a child already has rhinitis and cleaning up his or her room leads to no improvement, the child should be taken for medical diagnosis and treatment. How long to wait to take this step depends on how uncomfortable the child is and whether there is any improvement. With moderately severe symptoms, one should not wait more than a few days to two weeks. With intermittent or very mild symptoms, a slightly longer delay will probably do no harm, but you should not let any physical discomfort drag on for months without getting a diagnosis.

Ongoing symptoms warrant diagnosis and treatment. What parents may describe as "just" an allergy or "only" a cold may be more serious. Among the possible underlying causes of continuing rhinitis is a sinus infection.

In the first three months of life, a stuffy nose and nasal discharge may be due to a congenital defect (choanal atresia). This is usually spotted in the hospital just after the baby is born, or by the child's pediatrician. Still, parents should be aware of it. The defect can usually be completely corrected by surgery.

Toddlers often stuff things up their noses. The result can be a smelly discharge from the affected nostril.

In apparent cases of asthma or rhinitis, it is also important to rule out cystic fibrosis. There is an understandable inclination among some parents to assume that a child cannot be seriously sick, and to avoid even thinking about such a disease that is not curable, which is the situation now with cystic fibrosis. But there is important work under way in the treatment of cystic fibrosis. For example, a drug has been developed that breaks up the mucus that blocks breathing in these young patients. This drug (DNAase) is a version of a naturally occurring human enzyme. Some 30 years ago doctors tried to treat cystic fibrosis with a version of this enzyme derived from cows, but allergic reactions among the patients—probably to cow proteins in the drug—made the treatment impractical. The new drug is genetically engineered, using the gene for the human enzyme and implanting it in animal cells.

In the laboratory, gene researchers have cured the defect in cystic fibrosis cells taken from the respiratory tract and pancreas of patients. The cure was effected by using a virus to insert a healthy gene controlling cystic fibrosis into the diseased cells.

Whether the treatment will work in patients remains to be seen, but scientists are extremely encouraged by these results.

Hay Fever

Hay fever, or seasonal allergic rhinitis, usually does not appear before age three, because it takes several years for this sensitivity to develop. However, children who live in the most southern areas of the United States or in any tropical or semitropical region may develop pollen allergies in the first year or two of life. The pollen season is essentially year-round, and so is the hay fever. The more typical pattern in the United States is the appearance of symptoms between age three and ten, with the disease getting worse for about three years and then stabilizing.

Children with hay fever can be helped by cromolyn nasal sprays and by antihistamines. Seldane, which is a popular non-soporific antihistamine, is not yet approved by the Food and Drug Administration for use with children under age 12, and Nasalcrom is not approved for children under age six. But if a physician thinks it advisable, both may be used in reduced doses for children as young as the age of three, under the doctor's supervision.

It is important to keep in mind that in children the side effects of drugs not only appear at much lower doses but may also be different from the reaction in adults. All children taking medicine should be carefully observed and any changes reported to the doctor. Medicating a child with over-the-counter drugs can be risky. The treatment should be discussed with a doctor. When you are buying a drug, tell the pharmacist the age of the child who will be using it and ask if there are any warnings about which you should be aware.

If the recommended treatment is with steroid sprays, this should be done under the supervision of an allergist or ear, nose, and throat specialist.

After age five, immunotherapy may be undertaken, and, as we noted, is often successful.

Middle-ear Disease

A complication of allergic rhinitis and other respiratory ailments that can be very serious for children is middle-ear disease (serous otitis media). It can also be caused by chronic exposure to some irritant, such as cigarette smoke.

Serous otitis media affects 10 million children annually in the

United States alone; it is the commonest reason for surgery among children here and the commonest cause of hearing loss. The disease is most frequently found among children under age five, and may be hidden at that age because the child often feels no pain.

As discussed earlier, when hearing loss occurs as children are learning to understand language and to speak, the child may miss important steps in the development of language skills. This can lead to speech disorders and apparent learning disabilities.

Middle-ear disease results from blockage of the Eustachian tube, which runs from the back of the throat to the ear. In children, the anatomy of the immature tube makes it more prone to infection, with material entering from the nose and throat. What parents can do to spot this disease is to consciously look out for any diminishment in hearing, especially in an infant or toddler. A child's hearing is normally very acute, and if a child does not turn toward or otherwise react to sounds as you would expect, notify your doctor. In addition, your child's hearing should be tested at least once a year.

Treatment depends on the underlying cause of the disease (see chapter 11). One type of therapy designed particularly for children is the insertion of tubes into the ears to drain them. The tubes are made to be extruded in a year or two, depending on what the doctor orders.

Children who have these tubes must follow their doctor's instructions carefully with regard to swimming, blowing their noses, and so on.

Sinus Disease

Sinus disease can arise as a complication of allergic rhinitis or as an independent entity (see chapter 11). The most worrisome aspect of sinus disease in a child, especially one younger than age five, is that, like serous otitis media, the disease is often hidden. The child often feels no pain or discomfort. The main symptom may be coughing. Sometimes, following a virus infection in the upper respiratory tract, a sinus infection sets in, marked by a smelly, clear-white to green nasal discharge. Again, coughing is common; there is often a barking cough at night, with apparent bronchitis. The child may run a low fever and be lethargic.

Although doctors today like to keep X rays to a minimum, if no explanation can be found for coughing, fatigue, and so on, a sinus X ray may be recommended.

The treatment is the same as for adults (see chapter 11).

Asthma in Children

One of the great satisfactions of treating children with asthma is that so often we can help these young patients, many of whom are weakened and frightened by the asthma, to manage their disease and be as active as other youngsters. Asthma is a common problem in childhood, affecting at one time or another 1 out of 14 youngsters. About twice as many boys as girls are affected in early childhood. But as they grow, boys tend to go into remission and girls tend to develop the disease. Among teenagers, boys and girls in equal numbers have asthma.

With infants and toddlers up to age five, the most common precipitating factor leading to asthma is a viral infection. The fact that the asthma has struck at such a young age, however, does not make the prognosis any worse or better.

The viruses most commonly implicated are respiratory syncytial virus, rhinovirus, and parainfluenza virus—in other words, bugs that cause colds. Why these viruses in some cases cause asthmatic wheezing is not known, but it may be because of actual damage done to the epithelium lining the respiratory tract. Genetics plays a role in some cases, as the young patients are likely to have an atopic history (that is, to suffer from hay fever or atopic dermatitis, or have parents who have these diseases or have asthma).

Once the viral infection has set up the asthma, allergens, exercise, and other standard causes of asthma (see chapter 9) may become the precipitating causes of future attacks. It seems that allergies may play a greater role in provoking asthma attacks in children than in adults.

Among children, an allergy to cow's milk may provoke asthma, but this thesis is somewhat controversial. The role of cow's milk has not been fully delineated. Among infants, the risk, if it is there, can be avoided by breast-feeding.

Children who develop asthma and who also test positive in skin tests for allergies are less likely to outgrow the asthma than children who are not allergic. And children with both asthma and eczema are especially likely to be stuck with the asthma for most of their lives.

For the majority of children, the prognosis is quite good. In one large study of 400 children with asthma, the majority had a mild, intermittent form of the disease, and more than half of these were free of asthma by age 21. A minority of these with mild asthma continued to have the disease all the way into adulthood.

Of the 100 children with *severe* asthma, 20 percent were asthma-free by age 21 and 40 percent were improved by that age. The other approximately 40 percent remained quite sick or their asthma got worse.

In summary, the most severe asthma is the least likely to go into remission, although most children can look forward to recovering well from asthma. Still, asthma is a serious disease in childhood, and while we can help children cope well with it and even become athletes (see chapter 9), the overall mortality rate for young asthmatics is rising.

The reasons for this rise are somewhat mysterious. Air pollution may be a factor (see chapter 9). Also, there may be a link between the increasing poverty and poor medical care among children in the United States and the rise in asthma deaths.

One factor that we recognize as a danger for children with very severe asthma is depression, as shown in a study by Dr. Robert Strunk at the National Jewish Center for Immunology and Respiratory Medicine in Denver. If your child is both asthmatic and depressed, extra care and attention are needed. Causes of depression in children include a recent divorce or death in the family, substance abuse or violence in the family, and continued unhappy experiences at school. Depression might be caused by the asthma drugs themselves. Signs of depression are lack of interest in life and adverse changes in sleeping and eating habits and in school performance.

Diagnosis and Treatment

Reaching a diagnosis of asthma in children is ordinarily not very different than with adults, but it can be more problematic with children under age five, who are too young to take a pulmonary-function test.

Many different terms are applied to episodes of wheezing during a respiratory infection: "wheezy bronchitis," "asthmatic bronchitis," and "pseudoasthma." A common view is that three or more episodes of wheezing are adequate evidence for a diagnosis of asthma. Diagnosis is especially difficult in those infants with asthma who wheeze only when suffering from respiratory infections.

Sometimes, as with adults, a cough is the only sign of asthma. A history of coughing worsening after exercise or at night can lead to a diagnosis of asthma. The cough may occur and persist only after a viral infection.

In differentiating asthma from other conditions that might cause the symptoms, a doctor looks for somewhat different conditions than in adults. Disorders of the cartilage in the trachea, cystic fibrosis, foreign bodies aspirated into the lung, infections such as croup, and anxiety conditions are primarily of concern among children, as compared to adults.

The treatment of children with asthma who are older than age four is essentially the same as with adults, except that lower doses of most medicines are used. (See chapter 9 for more on the treatment of asthma in both children and adults.)

Younger children, however, often are not able to use the inhalers that deliver medicines topically to the respiratory tract. To open the airways, they are more dependent on oral medicines, including theophylline and beta 2 agonists (Proventil, Ventolin, Alupent). Oral cortisone (corticosteroids) may also be needed.

Newly invented medication-delivery devices, such as Aero-Chamber and InspirEase, have recently lowered the age at which children can take drugs by inhalation from about age four to about age three, which is very helpful because of the undesirable side effects of the oral drugs. Another device, which consists of a nebulizer and a mask, can be used with children as young as nine months. Using such new inhalation devices, children can take not only the drugs mentioned above but also cromolyn sodium, which helps to prevent asthma attacks from starting and which must be taken by inhalation.

Theophylline, which is related to caffeine, may improve the attention span of older children, but a 1986 study suggested that it may cause learning and behavioral problems. This contributed to a reassessment of theophylline use that is going on today.

If you suspect that theophylline is causing your child difficulty, discuss the situation with your child's teachers so that they will understand the situation and report to you promptly if a significant problem is developing.

Theophylline is no longer considered a first-line drug, and you and your doctor may decide to reduce or eliminate theophylline, using instead cromolyn and inhaled beta 2 agonists (albuterol) or inhaled steroids. As it happens, once a child is old enough to take medicine by inhalation, inhaled cromolyn and beta 2 agonists are actually the drugs of choice.

Cortisone must be used with great care and restraint in infants and children. Among other side effects, it can prevent bone growth, resulting in short stature. Every effort must be made to use this drug in the lowest possible doses and for the shortest possible period of time.

Cigarette smoke in the house is bad for all children and especially for asthmatics. Areas your child frequents should be free of allergens, smoke, and other irritants that make the asthma worse.

As the child grows, your doctor should encourage him or her to live as fully as possible (see chapter 9). If the child's interests do not lie in sports, or in the very rare case that the asthma is too severe for sports, be sure to provide the child with other activities—art, music, reading, chess. Many great artists, statesmen, scientists, and others had to endure asthma in childhood.

17

Pregnancy and Allergies

Pregnancy should be a happy time, and for many women it is very happy indeed. The joy, however, may be tempered by considerable discomfort—from morning sickness in the early weeks to aches and fatigue near the end. This is normal. Even though some women feel wonderful throughout pregnancy, the majority experience stress and strain from time to time.

Ideally, pregnancy is planned, with health taken into account. Even before conception, the woman should try to be as physically well as possible, avoiding medicines or drugs that might undermine her health or that of the baby. Alcohol and cigarettes pose a risk to the fetus, even if only a slight risk in some cases.

If you intend to get pregnant, try not to indulge in alcohol, cigarettes, or other drugs from the time that conception may occur through to birth. You will have a better chance of avoiding a miscarriage and delivering a healthy child if you are completely drug-free.

Among smoking's destructive effects on the fetus is an increase in the risk that the child will develop asthma or other respiratory difficulties early in life.

If you take medicines frequently or regularly for any reason, and you want to become pregnant, you should discuss with your doctor how to manage medical matters prior to and during the pregnancy.

Among allergic diseases, the one that causes the most concern during pregnancy is asthma. But other allergies or their complications, such as sinus infections or skin infections, do pose problems for some patients.

Physical Changes in Pregnancy

The total impact of the myriad physical changes that occur in pregnancy, many of which are secondary to hormonal changes, can be difficult to predict with respect to allergies or asthma. With some patients allergies and asthma clear up during pregnancy; with some there is no significant change; and with some the allergies or asthma gets worse.

In pregnancy, there is an increase in the production of estrogen, which is believed to be related to the need for a larger blood flow to accommodate the developing fetus. The additional estrogen, however, causes changes in the lungs that tend to decrease the pulmonary exchange of gases. So this is a potential negative for anyone with asthma.

Another effect of high levels of estrogen is to slow the clearance of cortisol from the body. Cortisol is the equivalent of cortisone, which is used to treat severe asthmatic and allergic reactions. So in theory, having more cortisol should help people prone to such reactions.

The hormone progesterone, produced by the placenta in pregnancy, has among its effects relaxation of the smooth muscle throughout the body. The sphincter muscle between the esophagus and stomach therefore may slacken, with a greater likelihood of reflux of stomach contents into the esophagus. This, as we have noted, can make asthma worse in some patients.

To help avoid this reflux and the resultant heartburn, doctors typically advise women in the latter stages of pregnancy to eat lightly (several small meals per day rather than one large one) and to avoid very spicy and fatty dishes. Sleeping with your head and shoulders raised up on pillows or a bolster may also help.

Progesterone also increases the rate of respiration. The more rapid breathing (hyperventilation) tends to counterbalance the depressive effect of estrogen on gas exchange. But hyperventilation during pregnancy may cause a worsening of asthma in some women; the hyperventilation is similar to the heavy breathing that follows exercise, which in some people triggers asthma attacks.

All in all, the sum of the effects of estrogen and progesterone on respiration, especially in asthmatics, is not clear one way or another. As it happens, about one-third of asthmatics improve in pregnancy (especially if the asthma is mild), about one-third get worse, and one-third stay the same.

But any condition affecting respiration needs to be watched in pregnancy because of the increased respiratory burden in these nine months. The lungs must provide more oxygen for the baby and excrete more carbon dioxide. Similarly, the blood volume increases in pregnancy, requiring more work by the heart.

Hormonal changes also affect the lining of the nasal passages. The result is a condition known as vasomotor rhinitis of pregnancy. This causes nasal congestion, which is usually most noticeable in the last four to five months. It affects about one-third of pregnant women.

Because 50 percent of its genes come from the father, the fetus is, by immunological standards, a foreign invader, and it takes important changes in the immune system during the pregnancy to prevent the rejection of the fetus. All the means by which the immune system adjusts and permits the baby to grow are not known, but researchers have demonstrated the following changes, among others: a decrease in one kind of antibody (IgG); variable changes in the allergy antibody (IgE); changes in the numbers of white blood cells (some kinds increase, some decrease); and changes in the levels of the chemical mediators of allergic reactions, including histamine.

With these alterations in the immune system, one would expect dramatic effects on allergies in pregnant women. But as is the case with the total effect of hormonal changes, the picture is not clear, and your doctor probably will not be able to predict if your allergies or asthma will get better or worse in pregnancy.

Allergic Rhinitis

If you get hay fever seasonally, and badly enough that you would be very uncomfortable without medication, you might want to try to plan your pregnancy so that the first trimester is not in the hay-fever season. It is in these first three months that it is most important to take no medicines, or as few as possible, and only those that have been cleared as safe for use during pregnancy. Because the fetus is so vulnerable during this first trimester, you should consult your doctor before taking medication during a time in which you might conceive. Find out whether the medicine poses any risk to a developing fetus.

If you have perennial rhinitis or severe seasonal rhinitis, and anticipate that you would like to become pregnant in a year or so, you might consider starting immunotherapy. If you are a good candidate for this type of treatment (see chapter 6), it may be worthwhile to undertake it as a preventive, so that you do not feel the need for medicine during pregnancy.

A large study of pregnant women has demonstrated the safety of immunotherapy during pregnancy. But immunotherapy should be started well before pregnancy, not only so that the patient will have improved by the time she becomes pregnant but also so as to avoid the chance of an adverse reaction to a shot, less likely once a maintenance dose is achieved.

A woman who already suffers from allergic rhinitis may find that condition worsening during pregnancy. Recall that vasomotor rhinitis is a common condition in pregnancy, even among women who ordinarily have no such symptoms.

About one-third of pregnant women with pre-existing rhinitis experience a worsening of that condition. About one-fifth improve. Almost half experience no change.

A complication of rhinitis—sinusitis—is about six times more common in pregnant than in nonpregnant women.

Avoidance of allergens—that primary treatment in all allergy medicine—is especially important in pregnancy. Remove allergens from your home and keep allergens from making their way in from the out-of-doors. (See chapter 4.)

Safe and Unsafe Drugs

Although it is prudent to minimize medication in pregnancy, treatment is sometimes necessary. Infections should not be allowed to become established or to linger.

Many antibiotics are considered safe in pregnancy and are prescribed frequently and appropriately for pregnant patients.

Certain antibiotics, however, must not be used, especially tetracycline and its derivatives minocycline and doxycycline. Iodides, too, should be shunned.

Tetracycline, a drug with many side effects, discolors the teeth of fetuses and children, and therefore is not used in pregnancy or in children under age eight. Iodides tend to cause goiter in fetuses.

Certain antihistamines may be used, but with caution. Their use should be supervised by your doctor. PBZ (tripelennamine) is considered the safest antihistamine in pregnancy. If it does not work, the next choices would be chlorpheniramine, hydroxyzine, or diphenhydramine. Incidentally, once the baby is born, neither PBZ nor other antihistamines are recommended if the mother is breast-feeding.

High doses of antihistamines should not be taken, particularly near the end of pregnancy. There is a higher incidence of retrolental fibroplasia (which causes blindness in some premature babies) among women who have taken antihistamines on a regular basis and who give birth to premature or small babies weighing 1,500 grams (5.25 pounds) or less.

If there is a known risk of prematurity, as for example when there are multiple fetuses, then antihistamine use, if any, should be carefully supervised by a physician.

The only oral decongestant considered safe in pregnancy is pseudoephedrine. Among topical decongestants, oxymetazoline in a nasal spray is not appreciably absorbed and is probably safe, although there are no data to substantiate this.

One of the better medicines in terms of safety and effectiveness in treating allergic rhinitis is cromolyn in topical form (Nasalcrom for the nose and Opticrom for the eyes). The drawback is that this medicine is strictly a preventive and takes a couple of weeks to work.

The research evidence on the safety of nasal steroids is mixed. In animal studies, an effect on fetuses has been observed. The apparent safety of inhaled steroids in pregnant women with asthma suggests that the nasal forms are safe, except for dexamethasone (Decadron), which can be absorbed systemically. (See the section below on asthma during pregnancy for more information on steroids.)

With rhinitis, toughing it out through pregnancy without using antihistamines or other allergy medicines is often the best course. But you should also be guided by your doctor. Severe symptoms of rhinitis may warrant treatment, if only to prevent sinusitis or other infections. When drugs are used, topical medication is preferable to oral medication.

Asthma

The warning not to be overly strict in avoiding medication during pregnancy applies even more to asthma than rhinitis. The developing fetus needs a constant supply of oxygen through the mother's bloodstream. But as the fetus grows, it presses upward against the pulmonary cavity, reducing the volume of gas in the mother's lungs. So if blood oxygen is depleted by asthma attacks, the fetus may be deprived of some of the oxygen it needs.

The aim in pregnancy, therefore, is to maintain optimal oxygen in the mother's lungs. If you have asthma, treatment to maintain oxygen levels may be necessary, even including use of steroids.

Whether or not ongoing medication is needed, the outlook for the pregnancy is very good. It is essential, however, that the health of the woman and fetus be monitored throughout pregnancy by the appropriate doctors, normally an obstetrician and allergy or pulmonary specialist.

There is conflicting evidence as to whether or not women with asthma have a greater incidence of complications in pregnancy, including toxemia, vaginal bleeding, and (in the first trimester) nausea and vomiting, but at any rate, the increase in risk is not dramatic.

There is *no* increase in the risk of death from asthma during pregnancy. There is a *slightly* higher risk of the fetus not surviving to term when the mother is asthmatic and a *slightly* higher risk of premature birth, but the increase in each risk is in the range of 2 or 3 in 100.

For some people with asthma, it is difficult to distinguish between an asthma attack and the effects of anxiety or fatigue that mimic asthma symptoms. Making the distinction can be more difficult in pregnancy, because the increased blood volume and rate of respiration now and then cause breathlessness and a pounding heart even in the healthiest women. These sensations can be unsettling. Naturally you may wonder if you are having an asthma attack.

Discuss these changes with your doctor. If there is doubt as to whether the breathlessness is normal or abnormal, a pulmonary-function test or other lung assessment may be indicated.

There is sophisticated medical help available for coping with asthma-related problems in pregnancy. Asthma has been extremely well studied, with the result that many specialists (allergists or pulmonary specialists) have the expertise to guide the asthma patient. The outcome of any pregnancy cannot be guaranteed, but the authors of this book are among the thousands of physicians who can attest from personal experience that even severely asthmatic, steroid-dependent women can have healthy, normal babies.

Safe Medications

Ideally, if you have asthma, before conception you should discuss with both an asthma specialist and an obstetrician how to manage the pregnancy. If you can find a team that has worked together successfully before, all the better.

To minimize the need for drugs, avoidance of asthma triggers—whether these be allergens such as dust mites or cockroaches, or events, such as vigorous exercise—should be conscientiously attempted.

Another aim is to attain optimal treatment prior to conception. It is best when possible to rely on inhaled beta 2 agonists or cromolyn (Intal) and, if necessary, inhaled steroids rather than oral steroids—but it is not always possible. The appropriate oral steroids are prednisone and methylprednisolone. Dexamethasone (Decadron) should not be used. Even in nasal-spray and inhaler form, it may be absorbed and affect the fetus.

A cromolyn trial may be in order several months before conception. This drug has tested as very safe in pregnancy (it has a category B rating—see the chart below), and it can eliminate or decrease the need to use other drugs. But it may take up to two months to become fully effective, so you need to get started early with it.

Mild intermittent asthma can often be adequately controlled with inhaled beta 2 agonists, often in combination with cromolyn.

Albuterol is used most commonly, but in pregnancy terbutaline (Brethaire) has tested as safest. Next would come metaproterenol (Metaprel, Alupent), but there is probably not much difference between this and albuterol (Proventil, Ventolin). Brethaire gets a category B safety rating, and metaproterenol is in category C (see chart below).

The oral forms of the beta 2 agonists (adrenalinelike drugs) are less suited for use in pregnancy, and they have not been cleared by the FDA for such use. For one thing, they retard labor, and there are some other complications associated with their use.

Testing indicates that theophylline (which is related to caffeine) has a good safety record, but it does not rate as high as cromolyn on the safety scale (it has a C rating, compared to cromolyn's B). Many doctors are cautious in using it during pregnancy. A patient who is well controlled on theophylline may be left on it during pregnancy if there is concern she may not do as well on inhalers alone.

Inhaled steroids can be extremely helpful. They usually have a C rating. Data suggest that their use by asthmatics in pregnancy leads to no increase in the average number of fetal malformations or abortions (miscarriages), although data from animals show a slight adverse tendency.

The inhaled steroid beclomethasone (Beclovent and Vanceril) is absorbed only minimally into the bloodstream. It now has a category C rating, but may soon be upgraded to a B on the basis of recent human studies.

Triamcinolone acetonide (Azmacort) has a lower safety rating and probably should be bypassed unless you are intolerant of the other drugs. None of these drugs, however, has been unequivocally demonstrated to be harmful to the human fetus.

Even oral steroids can be used successfully in pregnancy, although the careful medical supervision that is always important with these drugs must be even more scrupulous when the patient is pregnant.

Atrovent, a form of atropine used to treat certain types of asthma, is also considered safe. It is in category B.

A word on the pregnancy–safety rating system: The Food and Drug Administration gives drugs grades, ranging from A to D, with an X at the bottom rank, based on trials with pregnant animals and humans. These ratings are not always as definitive as one would like and are sometimes out-of-date. Also, not all drugs are rated. But the rating system provides some guidelines.

The system is set up as follows:

Rating Category	Animal Data	Human Studies	
A	Negative	Negative	*Safest*
B	Negative	Not done	
B	Positive	Negative	
C	Positive	Not done	
C	Not done	Not done	
D	Positive or negative	Positive	
X	Positive	Positive	*Least Safe*

Negative means that when the drug was used during pregnancy, no more fetal malformations or abortions appeared than would be expected on average without the drug. During pregnancy it is recommended to avoid a drug with a D rating, such as Azmacort.

Eczema and Hives

Atopic dermatitis, or eczema, is rarely of concern in pregnancy. Nevertheless, because research with animals has shown fetal defects associated with the most potent steroid creams and ointments—as yet there is no evidence from studies of humans—it seems prudent to use the lowest-potency topical medicine that will work. If the patient has widespread, severe skin disease, it may be preferable to use oral steroids rather than lavish amounts of high-potency topical steroids.

Hives, or urticaria, with swelling (angioedema) also are not usually a major concern in pregnancy. Sometimes hives are triggered by an underlying infection, such as hepatitis, so of course undiagnosed hives should be seen by a doctor and diagnosed, before conception if possible.

About 1 woman in 100, usually in her first pregnancy, will develop an urticarialike rash around abdominal stretch marks. A mild cortisone cream often takes care of the problem.

The woman who suffers from frequent acute hives or from severe chronic hives should be supervised by an allergist during pregnancy. Antihistamines rated safe for pregnant women should be tried first, starting with tripelennamine (PBZ). In rare, severe urticaria, oral steroids may be needed.

The woman who suffers from urticaria triggered by cold may have to avoid cold during pregnancy as far as possible. The antihistamine ordinarily used to control the disease, cyproheptadine (Periactin) has a category B rating for pregnancy.

Delivery rooms and operating rooms tend to be rather chilly. So if you suffer from hives induced by cold, be sure that your obstetrician knows this. A special effort should be made to keep you warm during labor and delivery.

Angioedema and Anaphylaxis

A major medical concern at any time is angioedema, or swelling, associated with anaphylaxis.

Anaphylaxis, described in chapter 13, is a systemic allergic reaction in which the airways swell and close and the patient may go into shock and die. Naturally, the aim in pregnancy is to prevent anaphylaxis from occurring. If it does occur, aggressive emergency treatment must be taken. Delay or diminishment of standard treatment only adds to the danger for both fetus and mother.

Exercise-induced anaphylaxis is sometimes associated with particular foods, as described earlier. The remedy is simple in such cases: avoid the food, or better yet, avoid both the food and exercising for several hours after eating.

If exercise alone has induced anaphylaxis in the past, then exercise anywhere near that level should not be done in pregnancy. Apparently, the rigors of labor will not induce an anaphylactic episode, but the characteristics of exercise-induced anaphylaxis are not yet known.

Idiopathic anaphylaxis, which means anaphylaxis for which no cause has been discovered, is also very rare and not well studied. Patients who have had episodes of such anaphylaxis are sometimes treated with oral steroids, and it has not been shown one way or the other whether it is better to continue this treatment during pregnancy or abandon it.

If you suffer from either of these disorders, you should ask your doctor, preferably before conception, to help you find a specialist or specialized care center with experience in treating these disorders.

Hereditary angioedema, which can lead to throat swelling and death, is also a dangerous and rare disease, but better studied than the two disorders just mentioned. It tends to recede in pregnancy. In one study, 23 of 25 women experienced markedly fewer or no attacks during pregnancy.

The ordinary treatment for hereditary angioedema is based on the use of hormones related to testosterone and is not recommended for pregnant women. In fact, these medications are dangerous to fetal development in the early weeks, and any woman of childbearing age taking them should be practicing effective contraception. If you are on hormone therapy and plan to get pregnant, consult with a doctor on the best time to stop medication.

Because it is surgery, a caesarean section can precipitate an episode of severe angioedema in someone with hereditary angioedema. Prior to surgery the patient can be treated with plasma infusions, which will work to prevent such episodes. Local anesthesia is preferable to general anesthesia, since putting a tube into the lungs can trigger an attack. Vaginal delivery seldom leads to an attack.

Childbirth

If you have asthma or another condition that may require medication during and after childbirth, then sometime in the seventh or eighth month of pregnancy talk over with your doctor what medicines you should take with you to the hospital. Some women with asthma carry inhalers right into the labor room, but this sort of thing is best arranged ahead of time.

Your doctor and allergist should consult, and one of the two should advise the hospital staff what medicines you will take and who is responsible for administering them. The arrangements should cover caesarean as well as vaginal delivery.

Similarly, if you are going to be breast-feeding—and this is normally the healthiest means of feeding for both mother and baby—your doctor may want to recommend some adjustments in your medicines.

A discussion of potential ways that alterations in diet during pregnancy can affect the allergic status of the child is included in chapter 16.

18

Surgery and Allergies

Allergies rarely complicate surgery, and surgery is rarely needed to treat allergies.

Chronic sinusitis is the only allergy-related disorder for which surgery is likely to be recommended. You should be very certain before committing yourself to the operation that such aggressive treatment really is needed. Get a second opinion from an ear, nose, and throat specialist affiliated with a teaching hospital, preferably not the same hospital with which your original doctor is associated.

Anytime that you must enter a hospital or clinic for any surgery, it is very important that your doctor and the staff know of any allergies that you may have to drugs, dyes used in taking X rays or scans, and food. If you have a relative, friend, or nurse who will be with you in the hospital, this person should be aware of your allergies and watch what drugs and food you are given. Unfortunately, special notes regarding allergies are sometimes overlooked by hospital staff, even by doctors—maybe especially by doctors.

Allergic Rhinitis

If you suffer from seasonal or perennial allergic rhinitis, coughing and sneezing can complicate recovery from surgery on the nose or face (including, of course, cosmetic surgery), hernia surgery, or any abdominal surgery. Depending on the severity of your symptoms, it may be advisable to have elective surgery in a season when you can count on not being afflicted with rhinitis.

If you are considering immunotherapy, it might be best to get this treatment under way and your symptoms under control before having an operation. This issue of timing comes up fairly often with young adolescents, who tend to suffer from frequent colds and allergies, and a number of whom have corrective or cosmetic surgery in their teenage years.

If there is no sure way to avoid a flare-up of rhinitis or if the surgery is urgent, than consult your doctor to be certain that you have on hand adequate medication to suppress those sneezes and coughs. A series of sneezes or a hacking cough can open up a surgical incision.

Asthma

If you have asthma, it is important that the surgeon know about it, if possible even in emergency surgery. This is one more reason to wear a Medic Alert bracelet or carry such medical information in your wallet with your identification and your medical insurance card (which you can be sure hospital personnel will be looking for).

People with asthma are more than 20 times more liable than nonasthmatics to develop complications during or after surgery. The majority of these complications (75 percent) relate to the lungs. One out of 16 asymptomatic asthma patients develops wheezing during surgery.

The best course is to arrange preoperative planning between your asthma doctor and your surgeon. If a chest X ray has not been done recently or if your condition is worse, a new X ray may be needed. All asthmatics should have a pulmonary-function evaluation before surgery. If the surgery is a major procedure, a blood-gas test to measure levels of oxygen and carbon dioxide may be required.

Nobody likes a blood-gas test. It requires drawing arterial blood, which is often more painful than drawing venous blood as is done in regular blood tests. But it is very important to go into major surgery with good blood-gas levels.

Before an operation, theophylline levels should be assessed.

If you have moderate to severe asthma and are taking theophylline on a regular basis, arrangements must be made to continue the theophylline (in the form of aminophylline) via intravenous administration. In order to make a smooth transition, you may have to check into the hospital a day early to be sure that you are stable.

If you are currently taking steroids to control asthma or have taken them in the 18 months prior to surgery, your own adrenal-gland output may be suppressed. Not only oral steroids but also high doses of inhaled steroids may inhibit the adrenal glands.

Normally, the adrenal glands respond to the stress of surgery with a surge of hormone production. If your response is blunted, you may need steroid supplementation before and during surgery. This will be administered intravenously during the time that you are not allowed to eat or are anesthetized.

After the operation, these steroids will be tapered down quickly to your usual dose or to zero, if you can do without them.

The anesthetic gases used in surgery, such as halothane and enflurane, fortunately tend to dilate the bronchial tubes. Enflurane may be preferable for the patient on theophylline, because it is less likely to cause irregular heartbeats when used in conjunction with theophylline.

Some patients wonder whether their doctor will realize the danger if their asthma worsens during an operation. The anesthesiologist can monitor lung function and detect changes that require treatment.

When possible, it is best with asthmatic patients to avoid general anesthesia that requires insertion of a tube into the trachea (windpipe). But in some instances intubation must be done, and the benefits outweigh the risk of exacerbation of the asthma.

If you have asthma and still smoke, you must give up smoking before surgery.

If you are seriously addicted, ask your doctor for help or for a referral to a doctor, clinic, or program through which you can learn to kick the habit. Your local chapter of the American Cancer Society is another source that you can use for information on where to find help in breaking your habit.

Hives and Angioedema

Precautions for pregnant patients who suffer from a couple of very rare allergic disorders are reviewed in the chapter on pregnancy. Some of these apply to all such patients about to undergo surgical procedures.

If you break out in hives when your skin is exposed to the cold, a special effort should be made to keep you warm before, during, and after surgery. Your doctor and the staff should be aware of the problem.

If you lack C1 esterase inhibitor or if it does not function properly, special steps must be taken to protect you during both minor and major surgery, including oral surgery or even minor dental work. (Even the injection of a local anesthetic into the gums can precipitate an attack.)

The lack of C1 esterase inhibitor underlies the formerly extremely dangerous condition of hereditary angioedema (see chapter 12). People with this disease are prone to attacks of angioedema and in the past often died young. Today, the disease can be treated with male hormones related to testosterone.

There are two main means of protection when a patient with hereditary angioedema is preparing for surgery. First is the transfusion of two units of plasma (the fluid portion of blood) the day before surgery and two more units just before surgery. The plasma will supply the missing C1 esterase inhibitor. If the surgery is elective, treatment with androgens (male hormones) for one week prior to surgery should prevent an attack. If the patient is already on androgens, the dosage should be raised before an elective procedure.

If you are one of the few people who suffer from this rare disease, be sure that you are being monitored by a specialist familiar with treating the disease. A new drug is now being studied that may supply the missing C1 esterase inhibitor.

19

Questionable Theories and Treatments

Many times in this book you have been advised that the physiology of certain allergy reactions is "not fully understood" or is "not completely known" or is "not entirely clear." The immune system is extremely complex, and substantial research remains to be done to bring doctors to the point of being able to diagnose and treat all allergies and related immune-system malfunctions with ease and confidence.

Since allergy was first discovered, the range of symptoms found to be related to allergic sensitivity has been impressively wide, from mild sniffles associated with hay fever, to stomach and skin disorders, to the life-threatening choking of anaphylaxis. Given this variety of symptoms, it is understandable that allergy might be suspected as the cause of almost any unexplained ailment.

Most of us occasionally or even frequently experience mysterious discomforts that we cannot link to any particular infection, trauma, or other cause. These may be headaches, fatigue, nervousness, muscle and joint aches, and the like. It is not surprising that doctors and laypeople alike have wondered whether undiagnosed allergies are the cause of such symptoms. But what is surprising—at least to most ordinary doctors and researchers—

is that speculation about the role of allergy has led to an array of popularly accepted claims about allergy that are based on little if any scientific evidence.

In the last 50 years an influential nonscience of allergy has grown up alongside the main branch of allergy medicine. Called clinical ecology, or bioecology, this approach is based largely on unproven or unprovable hypotheses and treatments. Clinical ecologists include some doctors trained in allergy medicine and many who are not. In the latter group is a cluster of otolaryngologists. A 1983 article in *Consumer Reports* magazine noted, "Critics attribute this career change to increased competition for surgical patients."

The bad repute that surrounds clinical ecology does not mean that every idea put forward by clinical ecologists is unsound. Some of their concepts should receive and are receiving attention from research scientists. The problem arises when unproven hypotheses are presented as facts and consumers are induced to invest time and money on untested evaluation procedures and treatments.

Proof of a hypothesis in medicine usually involves testing according to scientific methods that minimize the chance of error. For example, there are statistical rules to follow: often a double-blind procedure is used, in which neither the researcher nor the patient knows whether what is being administered is the substance being tested or a placebo; and the study should be reproducible by anyone who wants to double-check the results. Indeed, before any medical claim is accepted as fact, the key studies should be repeated several times.

On some points in the theory of clinical ecology, there is no scientific evidence, or only disputed evidence, supporting the claim. On other points, the evidence is clearer: certain tests and treatments have been studied and shown to do no good. Yet they are still sold to the public.

Theories Underlying Clinical Ecology

In the 1940s, one of the pioneers in clinical ecology, Theron Randolph, suggested that maladaptation to the environment may result in a comprehensive "immune-system dysregulation."

Underlying this dysregulation is a hypersensitivity to several or many substances in the environment, often including food and water.

Typically, according to clinical-ecology theory, overexposure to one or more substances leads to an initial sensitivity, and this initial sensitivity flowers into a state of chronic or near total hypersensitivity to numerous environmental factors.

The substances that may trigger symptoms, according to clinical ecologists, are almost infinitely numerous: air pollutants; chemicals in building materials; food additives; many, many foods; synthetic fabrics; standard allergens such as pollen and mold spores; perfumes and aftershave lotions; water from most sources; viral infections; fungal infections, including excess growth of the *Candida albicans* organism; and so on.

The symptoms said to be traceable to environmental origins cover just about every problem a human being can have: behavior disorders; gastrointestinal discomfort; fatigue; depression; urinary complaints; sexual malfunction; hyperactivity; schizophrenia; respiratory difficulties; acne; headaches; arthritic pain; learning and memory disabilities; weight gain and weight loss; bedwetting; nagging cough; high blood pressure—and so on.

Even the symptoms of multiple sclerosis and cerebral palsy have been treated as allergy-related. Some clinical ecologists claim to treat food allergies with immunization. Mainstream physicians do not consider this an effective method for handling sensitivities to foods or chemicals.

The claims of clinical ecologists put mainstream doctors in a quandary. No one rules out the possibility of adverse effects arising from exposure to substances in the environment, including chemicals and food. This is a critical problem, and medical researchers in the past 20 years have made important discoveries relevant to it.

For example, in the 1980s researchers demonstrated that ozone (a common air pollutant in metropolitan areas on sunny days) has much more of an effect on respiration than had previously been thought. This finding is of great importance to asthma and cardiac patients.

There have been hundreds, if not thousands, of reports in the medical literature of exposure to chemicals leading to adverse effects on the skin, respiratory system, liver, and other organs. Most reactions are categorized as due to an intolerance, rather than an allergy. But a few chemicals, such as toluene-2, 4-disocyanate or TDI (used in plastics, foam, and adhesives), have been linked to allergic or other immunologic mechanisms. (TDI is associated with allergic asthma and hypersensitivity pneumonitis.)

As for adverse effects from food, despite numerous claims and warnings in popular literature, there is as yet no strong evidence that food allergies are a major health problem or have any connection to neurological diseases, such as multiple sclerosis. There is, in fact, no known cure, and the National Multiple Sclerosis Society is in constant conflict with healers and doctors, licensed and unlicensed, who use untested cures or palliatives to treat the disease.

In the four decades since it was first posed, no scientific proof has been found of the central hypothesis of clinical ecology: that environmental maladaptation causes immune-system dysregulation as described in the literature of clinical ecology.

There have been some reports that suggest that chronic exposure to certain chemicals and elements (for example, heavy metals and polychlorinated biphenyls) and perhaps even low-level magnetic fields can cause immune dysfunction. But this is not the extreme, comprehensive dysfunction described in clinical ecology.

Another general syndrome "discovered" by clinical ecologist A. H. Rowe in the 1940s is cerebral allergy. This is a kind of food allergy that affects the central nervous system, causing fatigue, confusion, irritability, depression, and so on. In one form or another, the concept of cerebral allergy continues to attract a popular following. But given the dearth of proof that it exists, treatment, in the form of restrictive diets or other measures, is difficult to justify medically or financially.

Another concept in clinical ecology is that maladapted patients develop an addiction to the substances to which they are sensitive. It has been suggested that a water-addicted patient should treat this problem by drinking from four or five different water sources each day.

Finally, there is the dramatic suggestion that there may be certain people who suffer from total immune-disorder syndrome. To borrow a phrase from Dr. Elliott Middleton, Jr., editor of a distinguished allergy textbook, these patients would be "allergic to the twentieth century." Such people are termed *universal responders*—they are adversely affected by everything.

There appears to be significant psychological maladjustment in the patients who have been described as suffering from this syndrome. Middleton notes that the methods of treatment used by clinical ecologists tend to promote phobic thinking, exaggerating psychological handicaps.

Middleton recommends further disciplined research into the possibility that such a syndrome exists. Unfortunately, such research requires isolating the patient in an environmental-care unit (ECU), which is an extremely expensive procedure. At the ECU at the Presbyterian/St. Luke's Medical Center in Denver, only porcelainized materials were used in the construction (done in 1979). The air is completely filtered. The water is unchlorinated. Organic foods are served. Elaborate rules exist to be sure that no exterior contaminants or subjective distortions confuse the search for factors that may be adversely affecting the patient.

Given the current extraordinary demands on the resources of medical-research funds, this line of investigation is likely to be limited for the time being. Nevertheless, use of an ECU with careful testing procedures does offer hope of pinpointing environmental factors that may disrupt the immune system in ways not previously recognized.

In the meantime, people should be aware that total immune-disorder syndrome is not a recognized disorder and that there is no reliable evidence as to what sort of treatment is appropriate.

The claims of clinical ecologists are essentially regarded as unacceptable by the great majority of allergists, by the professional organizations of allergists (the American Academy of Allergy and Immunology and the American College of Allergy and Immunology), by other medical organizations, such as the American College of Physicians and the American Medical Association, and by the Food and Drug Administration.

Immune-system Disease Related to Food

The only known connections at this time between diseases related to the immune system and the ingestion of food have little clinical application, although they are worth further study.

There have been a few reliably reported cases of a connection between eating alfalfa seeds and the appearance of an illness resembling lupus, which is an immune-system disease, or flare-ups of existing lupus. (More precisely, lupus is an autoimmune disease, which means a disease in which the patient's own immune system is causing the damage.)

In the early 1980s in Spain, contaminated cooking oil (the exact contaminant was never discovered) caused 300 deaths and 20,000 cases of a multisymptomatic disease with fever, cough, rashes, gastrointestinal symptoms, and blood abnormalities. Among the last was an increase in the level of eosinophils in the blood, a type of blood cell often elevated in patients with allergies and other immunological disorders.

Later some of these patients developed an illness resembling scleroderma, an autoimmune disease with multiple organ involvement. Certain patients were more at risk than others, and genetic analysis revealed that these people were also more at risk of developing other autoimmune diseases such as lupus or rheumatoid arthritis.

In 1989, it was recognized that the dietary supplement tryptophan (or at least some sources of it) could cause a serious disease characterized by muscle pain and high eosinophil counts. Tryptophan, an amino acid, is present naturally in most foods, especially meat, fish, poultry, and some cheeses, and seems to be harmless. Whether there was a contaminant in the pills or whether an altered form of tryptophan caused the illness is still not known.

These fairly recent discoveries, which are of interest to research scientists, may eventually lead to useful insights into links between certain foods or additives and autoimmune diseases. Clinical ecologists, however, are not particularly interested in studying or treating such diseases. The only exception would be rheumatoid arthritis, which has been treated with just about every legitimate and illegitimate therapy the human mind has been able to devise. Food allergy has been suggested as a cause, and complicated diets are sometimes prescribed by doctors of marginal status as arthritis experts.

But in fact, only on rare occasions has the removal of a food been shown to ameliorate the symptoms of rheumatoid arthritis. Both the cause and cure of this arthritis remain to be discovered, and by far the best course for the patient is to follow the therapy prescribed by a specialist in the disease, which can often alleviate its effects.

Questionable Tests and Treatments

Presently, a number of questionable testing methods for allergies are being marketed and recommended to the public. Many are associated with the clinical-ecology approach.

Some irresponsible doctors give patients expensive, esoteric tests of immune function that are not relevant to their symptoms, along with various marginal or useless tests and perhaps some standard tests as well. Exorbitant prices are charged for the evaluation, to say nothing of the treatment. Unfortunately, such abuses are not rare, and many of the physicians implicated are involved in ongoing legal battles with state health authorities and medical organizations.

Cytotoxic Testing

Testing for and diagnosing food allergies is frequently a difficult, frustrating process. Not surprisingly, therefore, a number of questionable tests are directed toward food allergies.

One of these procedures, cytotoxic leukocyte (white blood cell) testing, was excluded from Medicare and other insurance coverage in the 1980s for lack of proof that it is effective. The test kits have been outlawed by the Food and Drug Administration.

Cytotoxic leukocyte testing is based on the idea that there will be changes in a patient's leukocytes or a drop in their count after exposure to a food or other substance to which the patient is allergic. The test can be done in vivo, by exposing the patient to the substance and then drawing blood, or in vitro, by mixing the suspected substance with a blood sample. The latter method is more convenient and more widely used. Neither will be reliable. Consumers should avoid these tests and the doctors or other practitioners who advocate them.

Food Immune Complex Assay

This is another blood test designed to detect "hidden" food allergies. A measure is made of food immune complexes (antibodies coupled with food antigens) in the patient's serum. But actually food immune complexes cannot be correlated with any known disease and appear to be present normally.

Although there may be some future insight to be derived from this line of research, as of now absolutely no useful information can be obtained from this assay.

Intradermal Titration for Inhalant Allergens

Some early allergists, including H. Rinkel, believed that intradermal injection of inhalant allergens (such as pollen or dander) in varying strengths would not only reveal existing allergies but also determine an optimal dosage (the lowest effective dosage producing symptoms) for treating these allergies through immunotherapy. Unfortunately, the Rinkel method results in treatment with very low doses, which does not work. Higher doses are needed to attain immunity.

Intradermal Provocation Technique

The intradermal provocation technique is an adaptation of the Rinkel method used to detect food allergies. Long regarded as useless, it was decisively discredited in an article in the August 1990 issue of the *New England Journal of Medicine*. The method is based on injecting food allergens into the skin to provoke symptoms, such as restlessness or fatigue. Once the alleged allergy and an optimal dosage level has been identified, then further food injections once or twice a week are used to neutralize the response.

The research published in the *New England Journal of Medicine* found that, statistically, subjects could not distinguish between injections of placebo and injections of food in terms of symptoms produced or in terms of diminishing the supposed allergy. Moreover, intradermal injection of food can be dangerous. One might be dealing with a patient with a genuine food allergy who could suffer an overwhelming anaphylactic reaction.

Sublingual Provocation and Neutralization

The sublingual provocation and neutralization approach to testing and treatment is similar to that just described above, except that drops of food extracts are placed under the tongue. The neutralizing doses are also administered sublingually.

Defenders of this approach sometimes point to penicillin desensitization, which is occasionally successfully done in emer-

Allergies

gency situations through sublingual administrations of carefully regulated doses of the drug. But intermittent sublingual administration of food drops has been studied and does not have any beneficial effect.

Urine Autoinjection

Readers will no doubt be happy to hear that using injections of the patient's own urine to detect and treat allergies is not recommended. It is a useless and dangerous procedure that enjoyed a vogue in the 1930s and '40s.

Questionable Allergic Disorders
Yeast Hypersensitivity

The liveliest current allergy controversy is whether a sensitivity to yeast in the patient's body accounts for a multitude of symptoms, from fatigue to hyperactivity, headaches to flatulence.

The common yeast organism *Candida albicans,* normally present in the body, sometimes proliferates excessively, usually after a course of antibiotics that kill off organisms controlling yeast in most circumstances. In women the excess *Candida* may cause vaginal burning and itching, which can be treated with an antifungal drug. Around 1980, Doctors C. O. Truss and William Crook popularized the idea that excess yeast may impair the immune system, causing a general feeling of illness and symptoms that may affect any or every organ system. Particularly appealing was the idea that this infestation might account for otherwise unexplained exhaustion, irritability, difficulty concentrating, depression, and anxiety.

A craving for sweets and/or alcohol is said to be related to yeast hypersensitivity. Patients supposedly also feel bad on damp or moldy days, or when exposed to smoke or chemical odors.

The tests run to evaluate yeast levels include a *Candida* skin test and a stool test. These are almost always positive—they are so in over 90 percent of *all* people. The treatment is by medication to kill yeast organisms (usually the drug nystatin), as well as special diets and environmental controls.

Unfortunately, there have been no scientific studies to document the legitimacy of the theory or the efficacy of the treatment. Furthermore, in a study in the December 20, 1990, issue of *The New England Journal of Medicine,* the question of whether a treatment for the so-called Candidiasis Hypersensitivity Syndrome was effective yielded interesting results. Women with fatigue, premenstrual tension, gastrointestinal symptoms, depression, and other symptoms that fit the diagnostic criteria for this syndrome were treated with nystatin (an anti-candida drug used by clinical ecologists to treat the syndrome). There was no difference in outcome when a similar group of women were treated with a placebo (sugar pill). The authors concluded that therapy for such women with nystatin was unwarranted.

There is not ordinarily any danger involved in the treatment, and the placebo effect of finding a doctor who seems to understand and care can be very helpful. But on the other hand, some patients may be suffering from a viral illness or psychiatric depression for which there may be more appropriate treatment. Also, of course, the unproved treatment is not done for free, and some unscrupulous doctors recommend numerous additional tests and treatments of little worth.

As for the complex of symptoms including extreme fatigue, sometimes intermittent fever, and other often vague complaints, a more promising line of research seems to be to look for a covert viral infection.

Headaches

Many people, including some doctors, ascribe headaches to food allergies. But although sensitivity to certain foods does cause headaches in some cases, allergy is not usually involved.

Recent medical reports indicate that foods may play a role in some patients in producing migraine, cluster headaches, and some other headaches. It may be worthwhile for the patient to keep a food diary to see if the headaches and any type of food are linked. The following are the most likely known culprits: Alcohol can precipitate migraines and cluster headaches in some individuals. Migraines may also be related to tyramine in aged cheese, herring, liver, dates, and figs. Chocolate contains a related chemical, phenylethylamine, which may also cause headaches. Sodium nitrate used in processed deli meats, and monosodium glutamate often used in Chinese food may also cause headaches in some people.

Certainly, poor eating habits may result in headaches. But if you have a problem with chronic headaches, beware of the doctor who thinks exclusively in terms of food allergy as the answer. Headaches are serious enough to warrant careful diagnosis.

The first step is to find out what kind of headache you have. The classic migraine headache is not just a severe headache. It is preceded by an "aura," a sensation that indicates the headache is coming on. There may be disturbances in vision at this time, such as perception of a flashing light or shimmers in the visual field. The headache itself consists of a deep, throbbing ache, often behind one eye. The patient is extremely sensitive to light or noise while the headache lasts, and this may be a few hours or even a couple of days. There may be nausea and vomiting. The underlying condition in migraines is a widening of the blood vessels to the brain. Migraines should be treated by a specialist.

Other vascular disorders may cause cluster headaches, which are extraordinarily painful. Characteristically, there are long periods of remission and then the headaches come back.

Sinus headaches may be associated with allergic rhinitis or any infection that causes inflammation and blockage of the sinuses (see chapter 11). The pain may be over the eyes, in the cheekbones, near the tear ducts, in the teeth, or in the top rear of the skull.

High blood pressure may be associated with headaches.

Tension and disorders involving the joint of the jaw (the temporomandibular joint) may cause aches on both sides of the back of the neck and a bandlike ache around the head.

Severe headache may be caused by meningitis (inflammation of the tissue covering the brain). Associated symptoms may include fever, a stiff neck, and/or a rash.

Sudden, severe headaches may be a sign that a stroke is occurring.

There is treatment available for almost all types of headache, but a reliable diagnosis must first be reached. Sudden, severe headaches should be evaluated immediately. A trip to the emergency room is in order if there is no other medical help available. Recurring, severe headaches should also be taken seriously. Usually, a neurologist is the specialist of choice in such cases.

Hyperactivity

The popular notion that food additives or other elements in food may cause hyperactivity in children dates back to the mid-1970s and a book by Dr. Ben Feingold, *Why Your Child Is Hyperactive*. Recently Dr. Crook, one of the authors of the *Candida*-allergy theory, proposed that a sugar allergy causes hyperactivity.

Some people are indeed adversely affected by certain food additives (see chapter 7), and many parents have observed that sweets seem to make their children wilder.

New studies indicate that one reason some youngsters are overenergized by sugar is that it stimulates adrenaline production. But this is a transient reaction, and allergy is not involved. The cure is to limit sugar intake.

Hyperactivity is an overused label, but chronic hyperactivity associated with difficulties in academic work and social adjustment is a serious problem that requires expert evaluation. The causes may range from use of cocaine by the mother during pregnancy to frustration and aggression arising when a learning-disabled child is not appropriately diagnosed and helped. (Some students with learning difficulties are also extremely bright, which only adds to their restlessness and anger.) Allergy testing is not, however, a productive diagnostic tool in cases of hyperactivity.

Danger Signs

Certain types of treatments for alleged allergies may cause harm and should sound an alarm as to the physician's honesty. These are:

• Highly restricted diets. Most people are allergic to only a few foods, if any, and do not need to eat only organic foods, or only vegetables, or large quantities of red meat. Children and elderly people are particularly at risk if the diet is unbalanced or inadequate.

- Allergy treatments for symptoms that may indicate a serious health problem. These would include severe headaches, severe joint pains, chronic gastrointestinal disturbances, debilitating depression, and learning handicaps.
- Allergy or diet treatments for presently incurable diseases, such as multiple sclerosis or rheumatoid arthritis.
- Expensive nonstandard tests and treatments.

20

The Future

On the basis of work being done today, we can predict advances in the next decade that will help us better control and treat allergy reactions in a multitude of ways, from genetic intervention to symptom relief.

In the next five years, we expect refinement of our basic tools:

More effective, totally nonsoporific antihistamines.

More potent nonabsorbable steroid sprays, with fewer side effects.

Longer-acting sympathomimetic drugs (beta 2 agonists) that may be administered by way of a dermal patch. In general, dermal patches, which deliver small, continuous doses of medication, will be prescribed far more commonly.

Development of oral cromolyn-type drugs to block food reactions. Ketotifen, an oral cromolynlike drug expected to become available soon, will be useful in the treatment of asthma, especially the late-phase inflammatory reaction.

In new methods of drug delivery, look for breath-actuated inhalers. With these devices, the release of medicine is triggered by inhalation, and this increases the effective drug delivery to the lungs.

In immunotherapy, progress continues to be made in the development of purer, more standardized extracts. This will increase the efficacy of allergy shots while decreasing the risk of side effects. New polymerized extracts are expected to allow for fewer injections—fewer to reach the maximum dose, and less frequent injections thereafter (perhaps one every eight weeks). There may be safe, effective oral immunotherapy. Safe, effective immunotherapy may be developed for food allergies.

Both skin tests and laboratory blood tests should improve in reliability and complement each other. Eventually, lab blood tests should become so precise and inexpensive that they will be the primary diagnostic tool, with skin tests used for backup confirmation. Also, the blood will be taken from a finger prick rather than venipuncture.

Looking into the next century, immunotherapy might be reduced to one or two shots per year, providing total relief. The diagnostic method of choice may be as simple as attaching electrodes to your earlobe and taking a blood reading.

Allergists today anticipate the development in about ten years of a new class of anti-inflammatory drugs that will revolutionize therapy. These drugs will inhibit the action of the various chemical mediators of allergic inflammatory reaction. They should be useful not only in the treatment of allergic rhinitis and other allergic diseases but also in the treatment of asthma (whether allergic or not) and possibly also arthritis, colitis, and other inflammatory diseases.

Another type of drug on the horizon is a substance that will lock into the receptors on the IgE molecules. This new drug, a pentapetide, will latch on to the allergy antibody, taking up the receptors onto which an allergen would otherwise lock. In effect, this will stop allergy reactions before they start.

Scientists are also working on methods of limiting IgE synthesis, which would be another means of achieving the same result: arrest of the allergy reaction at the cellular level.

At an even more basic level, genetic manipulation may make it possible first to eliminate allergic disease in the newborn and perhaps eventually to change the genetic makeup of adults to eliminate allergic reactions.

Novel ways to manipulate the immune system will evolve, including use of interleukins to treat allergic disease. Already drugs that modulate the immune system, such as interferon, cyclosporin A, and thymic hormones, are being studied as treatment for atopic dermatitis. Photopheresis, a technique that involves exposing a patient's blood to light and thereby eliminating certain activated white blood cells, may find a role in alleviating severe allergic diseases.

In the meantime, with proper medical attention, the most serious and uncomfortable symptoms of asthma and allergy can be brought under control.

Appendix: List of Organizations

Allergists and Allergy Clinics

The following organizations provide information on allergists and allergy clinics. They also often have literature for the public on various allergic diseases and treatments.

American Academy of Allergy and Immunology
611 East Wells Street
Milwaukee, WI 53202
(414) 272-6071
Physician's Referral and Information Line: (800) 822-ASMA
    (2762)

National Institute of Allergy and Infectious Diseases
Office of Communications
9000 Rockville Pike
Bethesda, MD 20892
(301) 496-5717

American College of Allergy and Immunology
800 East Northwest Highway
Palatine, IL 60067
(312) 359-2800
(800) 842-7777

National Jewish Center for Immunology and Respiratory
  Medicine
1400 Jackson Street
Denver, CO 80206
(800) 222-LUNG (5864)

Asthma and Asthma Clinics

Sources of information on asthma and on clinics that specialize
in asthma:

American Academy of Allergy and Immunology
611 East Wells Street
Milwaukee, WI 53202
(800) 822-ASMA

American Lung Association
1740 Broadway
New York, NY 10019
(212) 315-8700

Asthma and Allergy Foundation of America
Suite 502
1125 15th Street, N.W.
Washington, DC 20005
(202) 466-7643
(800) 7ASTHMA (7278462)

National Asthma Education Program
4733 Bethesda Avenue
Bethesda, MD 20815
(301) 951-3260

National Jewish Center for Immunology and Respiratory Medicine (formerly National Jewish Hospital/National Asthma
  Center)
1400 Jackson Street
Denver, CO 80206
(800) 222-5864

American College of Allergy and Immunology
800 East Northwest Highway
Palatine, IL 60067
(312) 359-2800
(800) 842-7777

How to Use Metered Dose Inhaler (MDI)

This little pressurized metal container contains medications for treating and/or preventing asthma.
　How to use your MDI:

(1) Shake the MDI vigorously or you may not get the proper dose of medication.

(2) Depending on your doctor's advice, either hold the canister mouthpiece about 2 inches from your open mouth or in your mouth with your lips sealed around it. (If you are using a spacer that accomplishes the same effect as the 2-inch distance, then the mouthpiece of the spacer *must* be in your mouth with your lips around it.) Patients on high-dose inhaled steroids must use a spacer.

(3) Exhale all the air out of your lungs.

(4) As you start to take a deep breath in, actuate the canister to discharge a puff of medication and continue breathing in, sucking the medication into your lungs.

(5) Try to then hold your breath for 10 seconds before breathing out so that the medicine has time to settle in your lungs. Then resume normal breathing.

(6) If the MDI you are first using is a bronchodilator (and you should use the bronchodilator first if it is one of two or three inhalers being used at a given time), wait five minutes before taking the second puff (if instructed to take a second puff) or before using your other medication (e.g., inhaled steroid or inhaled cromolyn), so that your airways open up and subsequent puffs get into deeper airways in the lungs (the smaller airways that are susceptible to inflammation).

(7) The number of puffs to be used of each medication is as prescribed by your doctor. If you need more puffs of your bronchodilator or it is not relieving your symptoms, you *must* contact your doctor.

How to determine if your MDI is empty:

(1) Put 6–8 inches of water into a pan. Pull the metal canister from the mouthpiece and drop it into the water.
(2) The diagram below shows about how full your canister is.

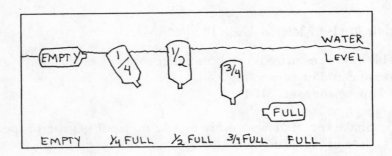

How to care for your MDI:

To prevent the valve from clogging with medication, rinse it with warm water every couple of days that you are using it.

TABLE A.1 COMPARATIVE COSTS OF ALLERGY TREATMENT IN THE UNITED STATES

	Denver	*Houston*	*Manhattan*	*Suburban N.Y.*
Initial visit (including comprehensive history and physical examination)	$100	$105	$200	$150
Average cost of allergy evaluation (skin tests)	400	400	450	400
Pulmonary functions (complete)	100	50	150	150
Allergy shot per visit, including serum costs	20	14	45	30
Cost of treatment for first year only for allergy shots	1,000	700	1,800	1,500
Cost of treatment for subsequent years only for allergy shots	500	400	1,000	750

This information was obtained by interview with one physician in each area who gave his costs and advised us that they were average for his area. These costs are circa 1991 and can change. They are meant only as an approximation as they have not been verified by extensive interview and research.

Adverse Reactions to Foods

Source: American Academy of Allergy and Immunology Committee on Adverse Reactions to Food. National Institute of Allergy and Infectious Diseases. U.S. Department of Health and Human Services. Public Health Service. National Institutes of Health. NIH Publication No. 84-2442, July 1984.

Food Groups

Researchers have found that if you are allergic to a particular food, there is a good chance that you may be allergic to other foods related to it. Table A.2 lists groups of food that share similar allergens; Table A.3 lists foods alphabetically and provides a group reference number so you can quickly locate and avoid related foods that might trigger an allergic reaction.

TABLE A.2 FOOD PROTEINS CLASSIFIED ACCORDING TO SIMILAR ALLERGIC POTENTIAL

Animal Groups

1. AMPHIBIANS
   frog

2. BIRDS (FLESH AND ORGANS)
   chicken
   Cornish hen
   duck
   goose
   grouse
   guinea hen (fowl)
   partridge
   pheasant
   pigeon
   quail
   squab
   turkey

3. CRUSTACEANS
   crab
   crayfish
   lobster
   prawn
   shrimp

4. EGGS (BIRD)
   ovomucoid
   ovovitellin
   white
   whole
   yolk

5. FISH (REPRESENTATIVE FAMILIES)
   Acipenseridae
     sturgeon (caviar)
   Anguillidae
     eel
   Argentinidae
     smelt
   Carangidae
     pompano
   Centrarchidae
     black bass
     crappie
     sunfish
   Clupeidae
     herring
     sardine
     shad
     sprat
   Cyprinidae
     carp
   Esocidae
     muskellunge
     pickerel
     pike
   Gadidae
     cod
     haddock
     hake

Gadidae (*cont.*)
 pollack
 scrod
Mugilidae
 mullet
Percidae
 perch
Pleuronectidae
 flounder
 halibut
Salmonidae
 grayling
 salmon
 trout
 whitefish
Sciendiae
 croaker
 drum
 redfish
 sea trout
 weakfish
Scombridae
 bonito
 mackerel
 tuna
Serranidae
 grouper
 rockfish
 white bass
Siluridae
 bullhead
 catfish
Soleidae
 sole
Sparidae
 porgy
 red snapper
Stolephoridae
 anchovy
Xyphidae
 swordfish

6. RED MEATS (FLESH AND INTERNAL ORGANS)
 a. Bovidae (cow)
  beef
  calf
  steer
  veal
 Gelatin
 Goat
 Ox
 Sheep
  lamb
  mutton
 Sweetbread

 b. Suidae (pig)
  bacon
  boar
  ham
  hog
  pig
  pork
  sausage
  scrapple
  sow
  swine

7. MILK PRODUCTS (COW, GOAT)
 butter
 buttermilk
 casein
 cheese
 cream
  sour
  whipped
 ice cream
 lactalbumin
 milk
  condensed
  evaporated
  homogenized
  powdered
  raw
  skimmed
 selected infant formulas
 yogurt

8. MOLLUSKS
 abalone
 clam
 cockle
 mussel
 octopus
 oyster
 quahog
 scallop
 snail (escargot)
 squid

9. REPTILES
 alligator
 crocodile
 rattlesnake
 terrapin
 turtle

Plant Groups

10. APPLE FAMILY
 apple
  cider
  vinegar (apple cider)
 crabapple

pear
quince
quince seed

11. BANANA FAMILY
banana
plantain

12. BEECH FAMILY
beechnut
chestnut
chinquapin

13. BIRCH FAMILY
filbert
hazelnut
wintergreen (*Betula* spp.)

14. BUCKWHEAT FAMILY
buckwheat
rhubarb
sorrel

15. CASHEW FAMILY
cashew
mango
pistachio

16. CITRUS FAMILY
citron
grapefruit
kumquat
lemon
lime
orange
tangelo
tangerine

17. COLA NUT FAMILY
chocolate (cocoa)
cola (kola) nut

18. FUNGI
mushroom
truffle
yeast
    baker's
    brewer's
    distiller's
    Fleischmann's
    lactose-fermenting
    lager beer

19. GINGER FAMILY
cardamon (cardamom,
    cardamum)
East Indian arrowroot
ginger
turmeric

20. GOOSEFOOT FAMILY
beet

lamb's quarters
spinach
Swiss chard

21. GOURD (MELON) FAMILY
cantaloupe (muskmelon)
casaba (winter muskmelon)
Chinese watermelon
citron melon
cucumber
gherkin
honeydew melon
Persian melon
pumpkin
summer squash
watermelon
winter squash

22. GRAPE FAMILY
champagne
grape
raisin
vinegar (wine)
wine (grape)

23. GRASS (CEREAL) FAMILY
bamboo
barley
corn (maize)
hominy
malt (germinated grain)
millet
oat
popcorn
rice
rye
sorghum
sugar cane
wheat
    bran
    germ
    gliadin
    globulin
    glutenin
    leucosin
    proteose
    whole

24. HEATH FAMILY
black huckleberry
blueberry
cranberry
wintergreen (*Pyrola* spp.)

25. LAUREL FAMILY
avocado
bay leaf
cinnamon
sassafras

Appendix

26. LECYTHIS FAMILY
    Brazil nut
27. LILY FAMILY
    aloe
    asparagus
    chives
    garlic
    leek
    onion
    sarsaparilla
    shallot
28. MADDER FAMILY
    coffee
29. MALLOW FAMILY
    cottonseed
    marshmallow
    okra (gumbo)
30. MINT FAMILY
    balm
    basil
    catnip
    horehound
    Japanese artichoke
    lavender
    marjoram
    mint
    oregano
    peppermint
    rosemary
    sage
    savory
    spearmint
    thyme
31. MORNING GLORY FAMILY
    sweet potato
    yam
32. MULBERRY FAMILY
    breadfruit
    breadnut
    fig
    hop
33. MUSTARD FAMILY
    broccoli
    Brussels sprouts
    cabbage
    cauliflower
    collards
    garden cress
    horseradish
    kale
    kohlrabi
    mustard
    radish

rutabaga
turnip
watercress
34. MYRTLE FAMILY
    allspice
    clove
    guava
    myrtle
    pimento
35. NIGHTSHADE FAMILY
    bell pepper
    cayenne pepper
    chili (paprika) (red pepper)
    eggplant
    ground cherry
    melon pear
    potato (white)
    strawberry tomato
    tobacco
    tomato
    tree tomato
36. NUTMEG FAMILY
    mace
    nutmeg
37. OLIVE FAMILY
    jasmine
    olive
38. ORCHID FAMILY
    vanilla
39. PALM FAMILY
    cabbage palm
    coconut
    date
40. PAPAYA FAMILY
    papain
    papaya
41. PARSLEY FAMILY
    anise
    caraway
    carrot
    celeriac
    celery
    coriander
    dill
    fennel
    parsley
    parsnip
42. PEA (LEGUME) FAMILY
    acacia
    alfalfa
    black-eyed pea (cowpea)
    broad bean (fava bean)

carob bean (St. John's bread)
chick pea (garbanzo)
common bean
   kidney
   navy
   pinto
   string (green)
Jack bean
lentil
licorice
lima bean
mesquite
pea
peanut
soybean
tamarind
tragacanth

43. PEPPER FAMILY
   black pepper

44. PINE FAMILY
   juniper
   pine nut (Pignolia)

45. PINEAPPLE FAMILY
   pineapple

46. PLUM FAMILY
   almond
   apricot
   cherry
   peach, nectarine
   plum, prune

47. POPPY FAMILY
   poppyseed

48. ROSE FAMILY
   black raspberry
   blackberry
   boysenberry, dewberry,
     loganberry
   red raspberry
   strawberry

49. SAXIFRAGE FAMILY
   currant, gooseberry

50. SUNFLOWER (COMPOSITE, ASTER) FAMILY
   absinthe (sagebrush, wormwood)
   artichoke
   camomile
   chicory
   dandelion
   endive, escarole
   Jerusalem artichoke
   lettuce
   oyster plant (salsify)
   safflower
   sunflower seed
   tansy
   tarragon

51. TEA FAMILY
   tea

52. WALNUT FAMILY
   black walnut
   butternut
   English walnut
   hickory nut
   pecan

TABLE A.3 FOOD GROUPS CLASSIFIED ACCORDING TO SIMILAR ALLERGIC POTENTIAL

Food	Group	Food	Group
abalone	8	artichoke	
absinthe	50	Japanese	30
acacia	42	Jerusalem	50
alfalfa	42	asparagus	27
alligator	9	avocado	25
allspice	34		
almond	46		
aloe	27	bacon	6b
anchovy (Stolephoridae)	5	balm	30
anise	41	bamboo	23
apple	10	banana	11
apricot	46	barley	23
arrowroot, East Indian	19	basil	30

Food	Group	Food	Group
bass, black		cherry	46
(Centrarchidae)	5	cherry, ground	35
bass, white (Serranidae)	5	chestnut	12
bay leaf	25	chicken	2
bean	42	chicory	50
broad (fava)		chili	35
carob (St. John's		chinquapin	12
bread)		chives	27
common		chocolate	17
kidney		cider	10
navy		cinnamon	25
pinto		citron	16
string (green)		citron melon	21
Jack		clam	8
lima		clove	34
beechnut	12	cockle	8
beef	6a	cocoa	17
beet	20	coconut	39
blackberry	48	cod (Gadidae)	5
blueberry	24	coffee	28
boar	6b	collards	33
bonito (Scombridae)	5	cola (kola) nut	17
boysenberry	48	coriander	41
Brazil nut	26	corn	23
breadfruit	32	Cornish hen	2
breadnut	32	cottonseed	29
broccoli	33	cow	6a
Brussels sprouts	33	cowpea	42
buckwheat	14	crab	3
bullhead (Siluridae)	5	crabapple	10
butter	7	cranberry	24
buttermilk	7	crappie (Centrarchidae)	5
butternut	52	crayfish	3
		cream	7
cabbage	33	sour	
cabbage palm	39	whipped	
calf	6a	croaker (Scienidae)	5
camomile	50	crocodile	9
cantaloupe	21	cucumber	21
caraway	41	currant	49
cardamon	19		
carp (Cyprinidae)	5	dandelion	50
carrot	41	date	39
casaba	21	dewberry	48
casein	7	dill	41
cashew	15	drum (Scienidae)	5
catfish (Siluridae)	5	duck	2
catnip	30		
cauliflower	33	eel (Anguillidae)	5
caviar (Acipenseridae)	5	egg	4
celeriac	41	white	
celery	41	whole	
champagne	22	yolk	
cheese	7	eggplant	35

Food	Group	Food	Group
endive	50	lactalbumin	7
escargot	8	lamb	6a
escarole	50	lamb's quarters	20
		lavender	30
fennel	41	leek	27
fig	32	lemon	16
filbert	13	lentil	42
flounder		lettuce	50
(Pleuronectidae)	5	licorice	42
frog	1	lime	16
		lobster	3
garbanzo	42	loganberry	48
garden cress	33		
garlic	27	mace	36
gelatin	6a	mackerel (Scombridae)	5
gherkin	21	maize	23
ginger	19	malt	23
goat	6a	mango	15
goose	2	marjoram	30
gooseberry	49	marshmallow	29
grape	22	melon pear	35
grapefruit	16	mesquite	42
grayling (Salmonidae)	5	milk	7
grouper (Serranidae)	5	millet	23
grouse	2	mint	30
guava	34	mulberry	32
guinea hen (fowl)	2	mullet (Mugilidae)	5
gumbo	29	mushroom	18
		muskellunge (Esocidae)	5
haddock (Gadidae)	5	muskmelon	21
hake (Gadidae)	5	mussel	8
halibut (Pleuronectidae)	5	mustard	33
ham	6b	mutton	6a
hazelnut	13	myrtle	34
herring (Clupeidae)	5		
hickory nut	52	nectarine	46
hog	6b	nutmeg	36
hominy	23		
honeydew melon	21	oat	23
hop	32	octopus	8
horehound	30	okra	29
horseradish	33	olive	37
huckleberry, black	24	onion	27
		orange	16
ice cream	7	oregano	30
infant formulas	7	ovomucoid	4
		ovovitellin	4
jasmine	37	ox	6a
juniper	44	oyster	8
		oyster plant	50
kale	33	papain	40
kohlrabi	33	papaya	40
kumquat	16	paprika	35

Food	Group	Food	Group
parsley	41	red snapper (Sparidae)	5
parsnip	41	redfish (Scienidae)	5
partridge	2	rhubarb	14
pea	42	rice	23
pea, black-eyed		rockfish (Serranidae)	5
(cowpea)	42	rosemary	30
pea, chick	42	rutabaga	33
peach	46	rye	23
peanut	42		
pear	10	safflower	50
pecan	52	sage	30
pepper		sagebrush	50
bell	35	salmon (Salmonidae)	5
black	43	salsify	50
cayenne	35	sardine (Clupeidae)	5
red	35	sarsaparilla	27
peppermint	30	sassafras	25
perch (Percidae)	5	sausage	6b
Persian melon	21	savory	30
pheasant	2	scallop	8
pickerel (Esocidae)	5	scrapple	6b
pig	6b	scrod (Gadidae)	5
pigeon	2	sea trout (Scienidae)	5
pike (Esocidae)	5	shad (Clupeidae)	5
pimento	34	shallot	27
pine nut (Pignolia)	44	sheep	6a
pineapple	45	shrimp	3
pistachio	15	smelt (Argentinidae)	5
plantain	11	snail	8
plum	46	sole (Soleidae)	5
pollack (Gadidae)	5	sorghum	23
pompano (Carangidae)	5	sorrel	14
popcorn	23	sow	6b
poppyseed	47	soybean	42
porgy (Sparidae)	5	spearmint	30
pork	6b	spinach	20
potato		sprat (Clupeidae)	5
sweet	31	squab	2
white	35	squash	
prawn	3	summer	21
prune	46	winter	21
pumpkin	21	squid	8
		steer	6a
quahog	8	strawberry	48
quail	2	sturgeon	
quince	10	(Acipenseridae)	5
quince seed	10	sugar beet	20
		sugar cane	23
radish	33	sunfish (Centrarchidae)	5
raisin	22	sunflower seed	50
raspberry		sweetbread	6a
black	48	swine	6b
red	48	Swiss chard	20
rattlesnake	9	swordfish (Xyphidae)	5

Food	Group	Food	Group
tamarind	42	watermelon	21
tangelo	16	watermelon, Chinese	21
tangerine	16	weakfish (Scienidae)	5
tansy	50	wheat	23
tarragon	50	bran	
tea	51	germ	
terrapin	9	gliadin	
thyme	30	globulin	
tobacco	35	glutenin	
tomato	35	leucosin	
tomato, strawberry	35	proteose	
tomato, tree	35	whole	
tragacanth	42	whitefish (Salmonidae)	5
trout (Salmonidae)	5	wine (grape)	22
truffle	18	winter muskmelon	21
tuna (Scombridae)	5	wintergreen	
turkey	2	*Betula* spp.	13
turmeric	19	*Pyrola* spp.	24
turnip	33	wormwood	50
turtle	9		
		yam	31
vanilla	38	yeast	18
veal	6a	baker's	
vinegar (apple cider)	10	brewer's	
vinegar (wine)	22	distiller's	
		Fleischmann's	
walnut	52	lactose-fermenting	
black		lager beer	
English		yogurt	7
watercress	33		

Bibliography and Resource Information

Books

Young, Stuart, M.D., with Susan Shulman and Martin Shulman, Ph.D. *The Asthma Handbook*. New York: Bantam, 1989. A comprehensive guide to understanding asthma for patients and their families. To order: except in N.Y. State, phone 800-223-6834, extension 9479. In N.Y. State, phone 212-765-6500, extension 9749.

Sander, Nancy. *A Parent's Guide to Asthma*. New York: Doubleday, 1989. How to help your child control asthma at home, school, and play. To order: Phone 800-878-4403.

The Allergy Cookbook: Diets Unlimited for Limited Diets and *Foods for Festive Occasions*. Allergy Information Association, 65 Tromley Drive, Etobicoke, Ontario M9B 5Y7 Canada. Phone 416-244-8585.

Captain Wonderlung. American Academy of Pediatrics, 141 Northwest Point Boulevard, Elk Grove Village, IL 60009. Phone 312-228-5005. An instructional comic book teaching breathing exercises for asthmatic children (in English, Spanish, and French).

Mendoza, Guillermo, M.D. *Peak Performance for Parents: A Strategy for Asthma Self-Assessment.* Order through Mothers of Asthmatics, Inc., 5316 Summit Drive, Fairfax, VA 22030. Phone 703-830-9320. Guide to peak flow meter use for asthmatics.

Parcel, Tiernan, Nader, and Weiner. *Teaching Myself About Asthma.* Health Education Associates, 14 N. Lake Road, Columbia, SC 29223. Phone 803-765-9233. A workbook for children.

Newsletters

Allergy News. Suite #150, 27800 Medical Center Road, Mission Viejo, CA 92691. Phone 714-364-2900. Written by two physicians for their patients. Available free to anyone.

Asthma Update. David C. Jamison, Editor, 123 Monticello Avenue, Annapolis, MD 21401. Comes out every three months and reviews the medical literature for new information about asthma.

MA Report. Nancy Sander, Editor, Suite 200, 3554 Chainbridge Road, Fairfax, VA 22030. Phone 800-878-4403. Published by Mother of Asthmatics, Inc. Useful information for parents of asthmatic children.

Organizations/Support Groups

Note: Many of these organizations have local, regional, or state chapters. Check your phone book.

Allentown Asthma and Allergy Support Group
923 Turner Street
Emmaus, PA 18049

American Academy of Allergy and Immunology
4th Floor
611 East Wells Street
Milwaukee, WI 53202
414-272-6071, 800-822-2762

American College of Allergy and Immunology
Executive Offices
Suite 1080
800 East Northwest Highway
Palatine, IL 60067
312-359-2800, 800-842-7777

American Lung Association
1740 Broadway
New York, NY 10019
212-315-8700

Association for the Care of Children's Health
3615 Wisconsin Avenue, N.W.
Washington, DC 20016
202-244-1801

Asthma and Allergy Foundation of America
Suite 502
1125 15th Street, N.W.
Washington, DC 20005
202-466-7643
800-727-8462

Florida State Chapter
Asthma and Allergy Foundation of America
1402 Dee Ann Drive
Brandon, FL 33511
813-684-3663

Mothers of Asthmatics, Inc.
Suite 200
3554 Chainbridge Road
Fairfax, VA 22030
800-878-4403

National Foundation for Asthma
Tucson Medical Center
P.O. Box 30069
Tucson, AZ 85751-0069
602-323-6046

National Heart, Lung and Blood Institute
NIH Building 31 Room 4A21
9000 Rockville Pike
Bethesda, MD 20892
301-496-4236

National Institute of Allergy and Infectious Diseases
Office of Communications
NIH Building 31 Room 7A32
9000 Rockville Pike
Bethesda, MD 20892
301-496-5717

National Jewish Center for Immunology and Respiratory
  Medicine
Public Affairs Department
1400 Jackson Street
Denver, CO 80206
303-398-1079, 800-222-LUNG (5864)

New York Support Group for Parents of Asthmatic and
  Allergic Children
201 East 28th Street
New York, NY 10016
212-889-3507
Queens 718-847-1148
Westchester 914-834-5852

Parents of Asthmatic Children
Greater Portland Area
6 Poplar Ridge Heights
Falmouth, ME 04105
207-797-9188

Parents of Asthmatic Children
1 Freeman Avenue
Denville, NJ 07834
201-627-6875

Parents of Asthmatic/Allergic Children
1412 Miramont Drive

Fort Collins, CO 80524
303-482-7395

Parents of Children with Asthma
9450 Preston Trail East
Ponte Vedra, FL 32082
904-285-5680
904-358-3362
904-285-1410

Sequoia Hospital District
Asthma Rehabilitation Coordinator
Whipple and Alameda
Redwood City, CA 94062
415-369-5811

Vermont Lung Association
30 Farrell Street
South Burlington, VT 05403
802-863-6817

Urban Asthma and Allergy Center
Suite 150
2300 Garrison Boulevard
Baltimore, MD 21216
301-566-LUNG

Summer Camps for Children with Asthma
Alaska

Champ Camp
ALA of Alaska
605 Barrow Street, Suite 2
Anchorage, AK 99501
907-276-5864

Arizona

Asthma Day Camp
ALA of Arizona
102 West McDowell Road

Phoenix, AZ 85003
602-258-7505

Camp Not-A-Wheeze
Arizona Asthma Foundation
5410 West Thunderbird Road
Glendale, AZ 85306
602-843-2991

Arkansas

Asthma Camp
ALA of Arkansas
P.O. Box 3857
Little Rock, AR 72203
501-224-5864

Camp Aldersgate
MedCamps, Inc.
ALA of Arkansas
2000 Aldersgate Road
Little Rock, AR 72205
501-225-1444

California

Asthma Camp
ALA of Los Angeles County
P.O. Box 36926
Los Angeles, CA 90036-0926
213-935-5864

Breathe Easy Day Camp
ALA of Alameda County
295 27th Street
Oakland, CA 94612
415-893-5474

Camp Concoso
ALA of Contra Costa/Solano
105 Astrid Drive
Pleasant Hill, CA 94523-4399
415-935-0472

Camp Discovery
ALA of Central California
P.O. Box 11187
Fresno, CA 93772-1187
209-266-5864

Camp Sierra
ALA of Central California
P.O. Box 11187
Fresno, CA 93772-1187
209-266-5864

Camp Superstuff
ALA of Redwood Empire
P.O. Box 1482
Santa Rosa, CA 95402-1482
707-527-5864

Camp Superstuff
ALA of San Francisco
562 Mission Street, #203
San Francisco, CA 94105
415-543-4410

Camp Superstuff
ALA of Santa Clara/San Benito Counties
1469 Park Avenue
San Jose, CA 95126
408-996-LUNG

Camp Superstuff
ALA of Superior California
2732 Cohasset Road, #A
Chico, CA 95926-0977
916-345-5864

Camp Wheez
ALA of Santa Barbara County
1510 San Andres Street
Santa Barbara, CA 93101-4104
805-963-1426

Club Wheez
ALA of San Mateo County

2250 Palm Avenue
San Mateo, CA 94403-1860
415-349-1111 or 349-1600

Running Springs
AAFA
5410 Wilshire Boulevard, Suite 1005
Los Angeles, CA 90036
213-937-7859

Scamp Camp
ALA of the Inland Counties
371 West 14th Street
San Bernardino, CA 92405
714-884-5864

Scamp Camp
ALA of Orange County
1717 North Broadway
Santa Ana, CA 92706-2675
714-835-5864

Scamp Camp
ALA of San Diego/Imperial Counties
P.O. Box 3879
San Diego, CA 92103
619-297-3901

Scamp Camp
ALA of Ventura County
P.O. Box 1627
Ventura, CA 93002
805-643-2189

Summer Asthma Camp
ALA of Long Beach
1002 Pacific Avenue
Long Beach, CA 90813-3098
213-436-9873

Colorado

Champ Camp
ALA of Colorado

1600 Race Street
Denver, CO 60206-1198
303-388-4327

Connecticut

Camp Treasure Chest
ALA of Connecticut
45 Ash Street
East Hartford, CT 06108
203-289-5401

District of Columbia

Camp Happy Lungs
ALA of the District of Columbia
475 H Street, N.W.
Washington, DC 20001
202-682-5864

Florida

Camp Superstuff
ALA of Dade-Monroe, Inc.
830 Brickell Plaza
Miami, FL 33131-3996
305-377-1771

Sunshine Station
ALA of Florida
P.O. Box 8127
Jacksonville, FL 32239-8127
904-743-2933

Georgia

Camp Breathe Easy
ALA of Atlanta
723 Piedmont Avenue, N.E.
Atlanta, GA 30365-0701
404-872-9653

Camp Superstuff
ALA of Georgia
2452 Spring Road

Smyrna, GA 30080
404-434-5864

Superstuff Asthma Day Camp
ALA of Georgia, West Central Branch
2546 Wynnton Road
Columbus, GA 31906
404-323-4700

Hawaii

Hawaii Asthma Camp/Camp Kokokahi
Aloha United Way
99128 Aiea Heights Drive, #107
Aiea, HI 96701

Illinois

Camp Action
Chicago Lung Association
1440 West Washington Boulevard
Chicago, IL 60607-1878
312-243-2000

Camp Ravenwood
AAFA, Greater Chicago Chapter
111 North Wabash, Suite 909
Chicago, IL 60602
312-346-0745

Camp Superkids
ALA of Illinois
P.O. Box 19239
Springfield, IL 62794-9239
217-528-3441

Indiana

Camp Superkids
ALA of Indiana
9410 Priority Way West Drive
Indianapolis, IN 46240
317-573-3900

Iowa

Camp Superkids
ALA of Iowa
1025 Ashworth Road, #410
West Des Moines, IA 50265
515-224-0800

Kansas

Camp Superbreathers
ALA of Kansas
1107 Parklane Office Park, #224
Wichita, KS 67218
316-687-3888

Kentucky

Camp Superkids
ALA of Kentucky
P.O. Box 969
Louisville, KY 40201
502-363-2652

Maine

Camp Opportunity
ALA of Maine
128 Sewall Street
Augusta, ME 04330
207-622-6394

Maryland

Camp Superkids
ALA of Maryland
1840 York Road, #K-M
Timonium, MD 21093-2120
301-560-2120

Massachusetts

Camp Chest Nut
ALA of Massachusetts

803 Summer Street
1st Floor
South Boston, MA 02127-1609
617-269-9720

Michigan

Camp Michi-Mac
ALA of Michigan
403 Seymour Avenue
Lansing, MI 48933-1179
517-484-4541

Camp Sun Deer
ALA of Southeast Michigan
18860 West Ten Mile Road
Southfield, MI 48075
313-559-5100

Minnesota

Camp Superkids
ALA of Hennepin County
1829 Portland Avenue
Minneapolis, MN 55404
612-871-7332

Camp Superkids
ALA of Minnesota
480 Concordia Avenue
St. Paul, MN 55103
612-224-4901

Missouri

Camp Lakewood
ALA of Missouri
YMCA of the Ozarks
1118 Hampton Avenue
St. Louis, MO 63139
314-645-5505

Camp Shawnee
ALA of Western Missouri

Kansas City, MO 64108
816-234-3097

Montana

Camp Huff 'n Puff
ALA of Montana
Christmas Seal Building
825 Helena Avenue
Helena, MT 59601
406-442-6556

Nebraska

Camp Superkids
ALA of Nebraska
8901 Indian Hills Drive, #107
Omaha, NE 68114
402-393-2222

Nevada

Camp Superkids
ALA of Nevada, Northern Region
P.O. Box 7056
Reno, NV 89510-7056
702-825-5864

Camp Superkids
ALA of Nevada, Southern Region
P.O. Box 44137
Las Vegas, NV 89116
702-454-2500

New Hampshire

Camp Superkids
ALA of New Hampshire
P.O. Box 1014
Manchester, NH 03105
603-669-2411

New Jersey

Camp Superkids
ALA of Central New Jersey
206 Westfield Avenue
Clark, NJ 07066
201-388-4556

Frost Valley YMCA
ALA of New Jersey
1600 Route 22 East
Union, NJ 07083
201-687-9340

New Mexico

Stephen Lopez Memorial Camp
   for Asthmatic Children
ALA of New Mexico
216 Truman N.E.
Albuquerque, NM 87108
305-265-0732

New York

Camp Superkids
ALA of Mid-New York
23 South Street
Utica, NY 13501
315-735-9225

Camp Superkids
ALA of Queens
112-25 Queens Boulevard
Forest Hills, NY 11375
718-263-5656

Superkids at Chingachgook
ALA of New York State
8 Mountain View Avenue
Albany, NY 12205
518-459-4197

Wagon Road Camp
Children's Aid Society

Box 47
Chappaqua, NY 10514
914-238-4761

North Carolina

Camp Challenge
ALA of North Carolina
P.O. Box 6176
Raleigh, NC 27628
919-782-2888

North Dakota

Dakota Super Kids Camp
ALA of North Dakota
P.O. Box 5004
Bismarck, ND 38502
701-223-5613

Ohio

Camp Superkids
ALA of Ohio, South Shore Branch
226 Street-Route 61 East
Norwalk, OH 44857
419-663-LUNG

Camp Superkids/Camp Libbey
ALA of Northwestern Ohio
425 Jefferson Avenue, #902
Toledo, OH 43604-1053
419-255-2378

Camp Superkids/Camp Mowana
ALA of Ohio
2276 Fleming Falls Road
Mansfield, OH 44903
614-279-1700

Camp Superkids XI
ALA of Southwestern Ohio
Room 400
2330 Victory Parkway

Cincinnati, OH 45206
513-751-3650

Oklahoma

Camp Breathe Easy
ALA of Oklahoma
P.O. Box 53303
Oklahoma City, OK 73152-3303
405-524-8471

Camp Green Country
ALA of Green Country, Oklahoma
1422 East 71, Suite N
Tulsa, OK 74136
918-747-3441

Oregon

Camp Christmas Seal
ALA of Oregon
P.O. Box 115
Portland, OR 97207
503-224-5145

Pennsylvania

Camp Breathe Easy
ALA of Central Pennsylvania
P.O. Box 1632
Harrisburg, PA 17105-1632
717-234-5991

Camp Huff 'n Puff
ALA of Western Pennsylvania
2851 Bedford Avenue
Pittsburgh, PA 15219
412-621-0400 or 800-553-1990

South Carolina

Camp Puff 'n Stuff
ALA of South Carolina, Coastal Branch
4970A Dorchester Road

Charleston, SC 29418
803-552-2851 or 552-2852

South Dakota

Camp Tepeetonka
South Dakota Lung Association
YMCA
230 South Minnesota
Sioux Falls, SD 57102
605-336-3190

Leif Ericson Day Camp
South Dakota Lung Association
McKennan Hospital
300 21st Street
Sioux Falls, SD 57105
605-339-7677

Texas

Jeff A. Green Asthma Camp
ALA of Dallas Area
7616 LBJ Freeway, Suite 100
Dallas, TX 75251
214-239-5864

Utah

Camp Superkids
ALA of Utah
1930 South 1100 East Street
Salt Lake City, UT 84106
801-484-4456

Virginia

Camp Holiday Trails
P.O. Box 5806
Charlottesville, VA 22905-0806
804-977-3781

Camp Superstuff
ALA of Virginia, Peninsula Region

732 Thimble Shoals Boulevard
Building E, Suite 305B
Newport News, VA 23606
804-886-5864

Camp Superstuff
ALA of Virginia, Southeastern Region
5349 East Princess Anne Road
Norfolk, VA 23502
804-855-3059

Washington

Camp Breathe Easy
ALA of Washington, Central Region
901 Summitview, #241
Yakima, WA 98902
509-248-4384

Inland Empire Children's Asthma Camp
ALA of Washington, Eastern Region
North 1322 Ash
Spokane, WA 99201
509-325-6516

Summer Asthma Camp
ALA of Washington
King County/NW Field Office
2625 Third Avenue
Seattle, WA 98121
206-441-5100

Wisconsin

Camp WIKIDAS
ALA of Wisconsin
1330 North 113th Street, #190
Milwaukee, WI 53226-3212
414-258-9100

Index